Massage is Weird

HOW TO BEAT BURNOUT AND KICK BUTT AS A MASSAGE THERAPIST

IAN HARVEY

Illustrations by Willa Urbanczyk, who you can find on Instagram @willa_drawzalot.

ISBN: 9798490647119

Table of Contents

Chapter 1. I Suck at Massage

You suck at massage? Hey, me too.

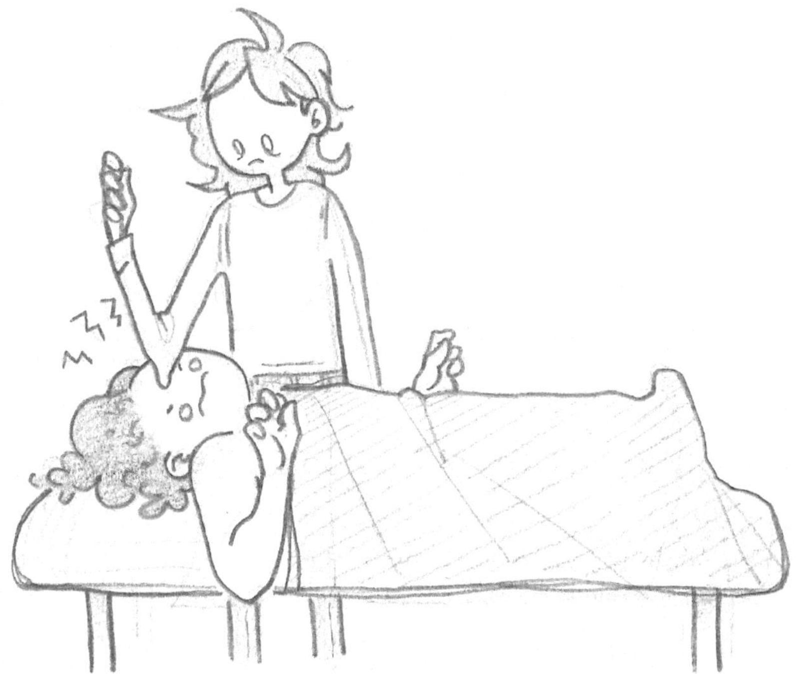

Or at least, that's what I say to myself every time I give a massage to a new client: "Well, this is the worst massage ever. No way they're rebooking. Would it be okay for me to stop the massage and just leave? I could slip out the window..." I find myself second-guessing my techniques, my flow, and the very concept of massage itself. It's one of the reasons I'm writing this book: Every massage therapist has doubts about their own abilities.

It's draining. It's demoralizing. And it's factually wrong. I've got good news for you – your massage is great, because *every* massage is great. Imagine things from the client's perspective:

- You get to just lie there.
- Someone is making purposeful, kind contact with your body.
- The person is planning to continue this contact for *an hour*.

- The room is mellow and the music is super chill.
- When all's said and done, your body feels good, and you might feel a little drunk.

Massage is pizza, and all pizza is good pizza. It doesn't matter if it's the frozen junk from the corner store or the artisanal masterpiece from the hipster place downtown, pizza is hard to mess up. You got your dough, your sauce, and your cheese, and as long as it's not burnt or covered in cat hair, it's going to be great.

Massage is amazing, not necessarily because of who you are or what you can do, but because of its ingredients. Patience. Purposeful contact. Kindness. If you've got these, it doesn't matter whether you hit just the right spots. Your time and intention are what make that hour worth every penny.

But I don't want to be "just good enough!"

That's understandable. We all strive for greatness, and we all want to stand out. For now, though, what would it mean to just be *pretty good*? Is that something that you could live with?

Let me spell out what it means to give a "good enough" massage: You've given an hour or more of your time to one person. You've contacted their body in a way that is accepting and nonjudgmental. You've made them feel like a whole person in ways that no other healthcare practitioner can. All of that is part and parcel of giving a "good enough" massage. That standard, no-frills massage can be life changing.

So, this isn't about settling. This is about realizing that your floor, the lowest you can go, is incredible. On your worst day, you're handing out transcendental experiences and supporting your clients in ways that no one else can. Let's say that you forget everything you've learned since massage school and fall back on the Swedish routine from your first month. You know what? Still awesome.

And *because that's your floor*, you can only go up from there. As much as I respect that gas station pizza and truly appreciate it when I'm hungry and don't feel like putting in a lot of effort to sustain my existence, there's something special about the hipster pizza place downtown. Maybe they have quirky names for their pizzas based on internet memes. Maybe they source their ingredients locally, or they have weird stuff like kale chips or quinoa. In any case, they put time into their product, and their love of pizza really shines through. When that pie comes out, it's a thing of beauty.

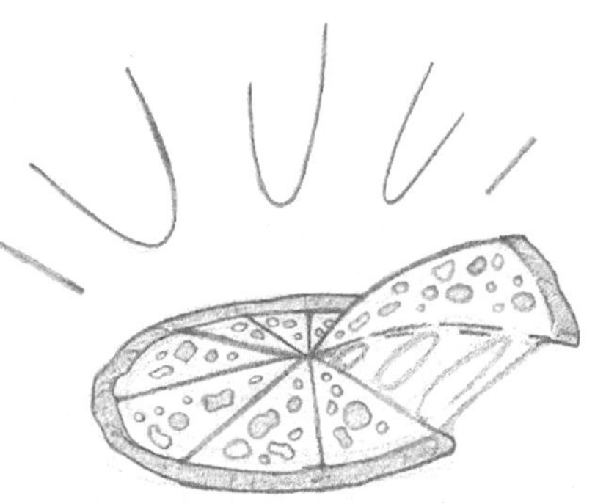

That's how I want my massage to be, and I bet you do too. You want your knowledge of anatomy to be self-evident with every stroke, and you want to tell a story with your hands. You want to contact structures that are relevant to your client's pain, and apply pressure in a way that says, "I feel what you feel." You want your client to be connected to their own body.

All great! I want this for you too, and we'll talk about how to achieve these things more as we go on. For now, though, think about what it means to just "be pizza." What does it mean when your floor, the lowest you can go, is pretty great and worth the money? It means you can't fail. It means you can experiment, and goof around, and try out moves that you learned in a weekend workshop (or just made up on the fly). It means that, even while you're thinking, "I suck, this massage sucks, I should just go home," your client is thinking, "ahhh, this is some good stuff."

On impostor syndrome

I was serious when I wrote that I still worry about how badly I'm doing, fifteen years in. As I give a massage I'll be wracked with doubt, wishing that I could just start the day over, or hand the client over to a better massage therapist. And you know what? That can actually be an indicator that I'm the right person for the job.

In psychology there's a phenomenon called *impostor syndrome*. It's not a mental illness, and it's not in the diagnostic manual, but rather it's just a pattern of belief and behavior so common that it's been given a name by researchers. Impostor syndrome is where an expert — a professor, a CEO, a master pizza chef — feels like they're a complete fraud. They go through their day wondering why they get paid so much and why people listen to them. They wonder when they'll finally be found out and tossed out on their ear. And here's the part that I want you to keep in your back pocket during those doubt-wracked days: These self-professed impostors tend to be the most competent and highly trained experts. Actual frauds rarely feel self-doubt; in fact, they can be some of the most confident people you'll ever meet.

In other words, if you doubt your massage skills, *that's a good sign*. It probably means that you're a legitimate expert, or at least on your way. It probably means that you're driven to constantly improve yourself. You take classes. You watch videos. You read books. You question yourself and your abilities, and you constantly strive to improve them. Impostor syndrome doesn't *cause* greatness, but it does seem to correlate with it.

So, massage can't possibly suck, not ever?

You want your massage to actually suck? Then get stuck. Stop growing as a massage therapist. Lose contact with the basics that you learned in massage school, and become really, really convinced that your way is the best way.

"Eh, I used to use dough when I made pizza, but I'm really into iceberg lettuce now. Throw some sauce and cheese on top and serve it cold. My customers love it."

That's not pizza, that's the worst salad ever.

So yes, I've had bad massages before, but it was always because they *didn't feel like massage.* The massage therapist had become convinced that they had found a better way: Lots of prodding, no more long flowing strokes, no more worrying about pain thresholds. In fact, let's get a quick top ten list going.

Top Ten Ways to Make Your Massage Actually Suck

1. Let your client get super chilly.
2. Dig into your client's "knots" until they're bruised.
3. Give your client a complex. "That's the tightest back I've ever felt!"
4. Talk the whole time, removing the focus from the massage.
5. Give inconsistent or unsatisfying pressure.
6. Stop your strokes short, losing your flow.
7. Forget about flow! It's time to start poking and prodding.
8. Ignore your client's areas of interest.
9. Ignore your client's preferred pressure.
10. Do the same thing over and over, hoping for the hour to finally, blissfully end.

For a massage to suck, you need to forgo an important component that you learned in massage school. Heck, if you can just remember these three ingredients, you should be fine:

1. Kindness. If your heart is in the right place, you can't fail.
2. Patience. Don't rush the process, and don't lose the bigger picture.
3. Communication. Speak and listen thoroughly.

If you've got all three of those things going for you, nothing in that top ten list will ever rear its ugly head.

But... I got a complaint from a client!

Okay, that's no fun. It has happened to me, so I might as well tell the story.

I was pretty new, working at a spa, and I had a head full of interesting new ideas. I didn't want to be your typical fluff-and-buff massage therapist, and I had come across some secret techniques. You see, I knew how to erase pain, just by working with trigger points that referred to those areas. Not only that, but I could work with those trigger points to relieve pain that people didn't even know they had! That's way more important than working with their areas of interest, or relaxation, or a holistic experience.

Because I was so awesome, I had started to change some things about my routine. While most massage therapists give full body massages, I knew that I could get better results by making the massage all about certain key areas. While most massage therapists use lotion or oil, I had found cocoa butter to be the best for the super slow, incredibly specific work that was now my specialty.

And, as you might expect when someone is giving a specialized not-quite-a-massage in a spa setting, a client wound up hating it. "He skipped my legs and my feet. He used cocoa butter, and I hate how that smells. It wasn't relaxing at all."

My first response was, of course, indignation. *How dare she?!* People love my iceberg lettuce pizza! Pizza dough is so passé, every *informed* customer wants lettuce!

Back in the real world: How was I supposed to know that she didn't like cocoa butter? And who cares about feet, her problem area was her upper back! I can't believe my boss is giving me grief about this, the rest of my clients love me.

Fortunately, after the indignation (and shame, and self-deprecation) had passed, I realized some important lessons, all of which relate to the basic ingredients above:

1. Kindness: I had stopped considering the whole person. I had started to cut my clients up into little bits that needed to be "treated" rather than just contacted conscientiously. I avoided

that client's feet because they looked a little funky to me, and I let my fear overrule my best practices as a therapist (more on foot fear later).

2. Patience: I had given up on flow and Swedish because they weren't "worth my time." In fact, I had become terrible at managing my time because I was so eager to use my cool skills. I would spend inordinate amounts of time with certain areas and skip over others, all without consulting the client.
3. Communication: I hadn't determined what my client expected out of that hour of contact. I didn't ask about my unusual massage lubricant. I honestly had no clue what her ideal massage was, because I didn't bother to have that conversation!

In the end, it was a great growing experience for me. Once I got over my misplaced indignation, I started reincorporating the relaxation techniques that I had begun to disdain, and I reconnected with the spirit of "flow" that my school had tried to instill in me. I never failed to work with the whole body without asking first, and I started spending more time on the pre-massage interview. As chagrined as I felt, I *needed* that complaint.

So, what should you do if you get a complaint? Take what information you can get from it, and then move on. Ask yourself: Was there something that I reasonably could have done differently? Could I have customized that massage better, especially in the presence of more thorough communication? Was I kind, and patient?

Figure out if something needs to change, and then get back to being yourself. Don't immediately discard your techniques or regimen (I still use some of those tools that I had fallen in love with back then), and don't lose sight of your unique style. If you encounter a setback, reconnect with your massage roots, redouble your communication efforts, and don't get discouraged.

And if someone just plain doesn't like your massage, or your office, or you? Then put them out of your mind, and don't feel like you need to chase them, or change who you are! People have different tastes, and while most people will enjoy your massage, some won't.

When there's a difference at a basic level like that, allow those people to migrate away without chasing them. Continue giving the massage that you find compelling and that your other clients love; some will leave, and others will stay. This process is normal, and it will gradually help you find the clientele that is best for you. You, in turn, will be best for them.

Giving up on judgment

So far, this chapter has been focused on the simple truth that it's difficult to actually suck at massage, and that it's a forgiving profession. There are a thousand ways of contacting the body, none of them necessarily more correct than the others. There are countless styles of body mechanics and ways of using your hands and forearms, all of which can be useful and successful parts of your personal practice. It's hard to go wrong, and even when you do, you can always make changes and corrections! Massage is a business where you can always reinvent yourself from day to day, and where the practitioner you are in March might be completely different from the one you are in September. Come as you are, take your time, and you'll be an excellent massage therapist.

As you consider this and what it means for your feelings of self-doubt and for your business prospects, realize that you can take it a step further. If you're having a hard day and you can't shake the feeling that your massage is bad and you should feel bad, I'd like you to try incanting the following magic spell: "Whatever happens, happens."

What if my massage sucks? What if my massage is great? What if my client's pain doesn't get better? What if it does? What if, what if. As my psychologist says, "what if" is the engine that drives all anxiety. You could spend all day spinning out imaginary outcomes, both precipitous disasters and glorious victories, and neither will get you any closer to achieving your goals or ridding yourself of your doubts. While realizing that your floor for achievement is naturally high and that the field of massage is forgiving can make for useful perspective (and perspective is great for making good decisions), the whole "what if" thing is rarely rational, and it doesn't tend to respond well to evidence.

So, try this: Throw outcomes out the window. Whatever happens, happens. Maybe your current client hates it, maybe they don't. Maybe that client who never rebooked didn't like your approach, or maybe they moved out of the area, or maybe they'll randomly be back in a year.

The same with pain and recovery outcomes. Some people will leave your office feeling better, others won't. Yes, you should look for patterns and try to refine your technique, but some people just don't respond to even the best medicine. You can't force it, even with the most incredible, next-level skills.

And, most importantly, realize what happens when you *need* for clients to come back, or *need* for them to get better. That's when we start sabotaging ourselves and engaging in behaviors that a professor of mine referred to as *grasping*, a concept he pulled from Buddhist psychology. This is where we attach an undue sense of need or importance to something external and spend a lot of energy trying to control what is ultimately out of our hands. People do this with love, and family, and finances. We get invested to such an extent that we start working against our own best interests. In love, this can be by driving people away. With finances, it's by throwing good money after bad.

In massage, we start *striving* for that positive outcome, often in ways that make that outcome less likely. By pressuring a client to return, we can easily push them away, no matter the quality of the massage. By grasping after that positive pain outcome, we might engage in therapeutically dubious behavior like jumping straight to very deep pressure, or using trigger point therapy to the exclusion of all else.

So, what's the alternative? Let the outcome be the outcome, and you can focus on the process. When it comes to client retention, use your best communication practices, and be satisfied with that. For pain relief, use the protocol that makes the most sense, execute it well, and make changes based on your client's needs. If that doesn't do the trick, you can make adjustments next session. If that client disappears, that's their prerogative.

Leaving impostor syndrome behind

Earlier in this chapter I wrote that you're likely to be exceptional *for the same reason* that you have impostor syndrome. You don't identify yourself as some all-knowing expert, so you watch videos, you trade techniques, you read books, and you keep pushing forward. Just realize that your learning drive is part of you, and that you can hang onto that while leaving the impostor syndrome in the nearest toxic waste barrel. By easing up on your attachment to outcomes, you're keeping the best parts of yourself, and the best parts of massage, while giving up on needless self-abuse.

If you're like me, some days will still be bad. Some days will still be filled with negative self-talk and self-sabotage, and you'll go home demoralized and exhausted. In those moments, be kind to yourself. Consider stepping away from outcomes for yourself as well. Maybe you'll overcome self-doubt, maybe you won't. Just do your best, invest in the process, and know that this will get you closer to your goals than grasping for perfection.

Chapter 2. I Suck at Deep Tissue

Deep tissue massage. Scary stuff. When you think of deep tissue, you might think of sinking your elbow through layers of muscle. You might think of stripping connective tissue until it's looser or breaking up adhesions. You might even think of moving fascia around – making it longer in some places, helping it move more freely in others. In other words, you might think of *fixing*.

I remember what it was like being a new massage therapist. I had so many powerful tools, capable of changing how a person walked, changing how comfortable they felt in their own body. As I learned more about anatomy and kinesiology, I started feeling like I had x-ray vision. I'd go to the gym and see poor souls, hunched over a machine, certainly hurting their own backs. "If only they'd maintain their lumbar curvature." I'd see a person with slumped posture and think, "they must have such tight pecs."

Then I'd think, "Just give me 30 minutes and I could fix it all!" After all, I had seen some amazing transformations in the classroom, and I had read plenty of books where the author described miraculous recoveries from chronic pain. Postures fixed! Backs healed! Frozen shoulders thawed!

The massage therapist as mechanic

This is a seductive philosophy, and it's one that really sucked me in at first. There was a heady confidence that came with knowing the *real* way to deal with pain, and how to easily treat conditions that doctors seemed so inept at handling. And you know what? I was wrong. Not only was I wrong, but I was putting way too much pressure on myself.

Let's deal with the "mechanic" myth. I see it a lot when dealing with different massage modalities and gurus. The thinking is that, if we can just balance the hips, or help the feet contact the floor, or align the spine, then everything else will follow. Pain will be resolved, movement will be easier, and we'll be treating the cause rather than the symptom.

This is all predicated on the idea that we can create long-term changes to the body in a single session. We release the fascia to soften and lengthen it, allowing that client to stand taller. We break up adhesions in long-abused regions of sliding tissue to allow new movement and less pain. We reconfigure the body to make it work better.

This, according to my clinical experience and my reading of the research, is incorrect. The collagen that we have been told to "break up" is stronger than the surrounding tissue[1][2], making our task impossible without inflicting trauma. Fascia, while invested with some contractile tissue, is not easily changed in a lasting way by short-term stimuli, but rather by long-term stresses like gravity and aging. If someone has a head-forward posture, this is a configuration they've earned over the course of years.

So I don't have magic scalpel hands...

What a relief. What a load off my mind. Let me tell you about what my process used to be like:

1. Start the posture and gait analyses the moment that the client walked in the door. Note any side-to-side imbalances, as well as any extreme kyphosis or lordosis.
2. Observe the client as they stand, again noting any imbalances. Does their head sit too far forward? Are they primarily breathing into their chest? How is their pelvis sitting?
3. Once they're on the table, make note of how the hips are aligned. Is one riding higher? How are their scapulae? Is one more protracted or winged than the other?
4. Start making corrections. If one hip is hiked, or if it did more work during the gait analysis, then correct it with stretching,

---

[1] https://pubmed.ncbi.nlm.nih.gov/23746520/
[2] https://pubmed.ncbi.nlm.nih.gov/25831858/

stripping, and myofascial release. Repeat with any other anomaly.

5. Reevaluate. Check the levels of the posterior superior iliac spines. See if the sacrum is lying flatter.
6. Maybe do some relaxing junk, if there's time.

I'm not going to lie, I'm exhausted just writing all of that. I hope you didn't abandon the list halfway through, or start using the pages for origami practice (though I hear that's really therapeutic).

I also hope I haven't alienated any of my readers. After all, many of you will have learned about posture analysis and correction in school, and you will have implemented it to positive effect. While there's some evidence that massage can affect posture[3], there's currently no reason to believe that we can *direct* that process.

Allow me to repeat: What a relief.

Imagine if we could use stretching and stripping to permanently change resting muscle length based on our designs. We could use our massage powers for evil, creating clients who are permanently bent to one side, one arm akimbo and the other out like an airplane wing. They would lope with one foot inverted and the other flat, one hip a full inch higher than the other!

Now, let the sheer ridiculousness of that sink in. We can't create massage monsters. For better or for worse, that also means that we can't rebalance the hips as if we were turning a screw or replacing a spring. Certainly not in a single session, and not without the client's nervous system being on board.

[3] https://pubmed.ncbi.nlm.nih.gov/26863146/

If I can't fix people, what can I do? Can I change anything?

You *can* change things. You can help people stop hurting. But it's not necessarily through any permanent change to their musculature or connective tissue, and it's not by retraining how their muscles fire. It's through an act of partnership with your client. It's by harnessing homeostasis.

You might remember homeostasis from massage school, or maybe biology class before that. It's the state of balance that a living system reaches between states of imbalance. Maybe your blood returns to its normal pH after a short bout of acidosis, or your heart rate drops back to 75 BPM after you go for a jog.

Pain and dysfunction can be considered states of imbalance. If you're seeing a client with chronic right shoulder pain, it's likely that they've irritated structures for years through repetitive motions and tension. If you go in with a "fixing" mindset, you might want to strip out the tight muscles and activate the slack ones. You may want to "clear a path" for impinged nerves, and flush away stagnant lymph.

What if, instead, you just gave the client and their body a lot of interesting stimuli, from lots of different angles? What might their body do with all that new information? Hopefully, it will do what bodies do best: Return to homeostasis.

Allowing change

You may have heard this from massage therapists before: "I don't fix people, I just create a space for change." Hippie nonsense! If they knew what they were doing, they'd dig in and break those adhesions!

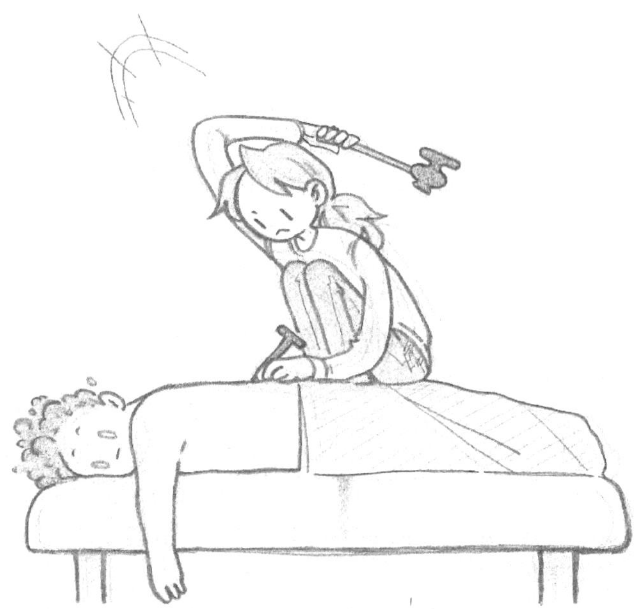

Whoa there, past me. That's not nonsense. The human body is actually exceptionally good at finding homeostasis, *given the right inputs*.

Imagine what your typical client with chronic upper back pain goes through. Day in and day out, for 8+ hours, they're hunched over a project. It might be a computer, or a head of hair, or a body that they're massaging. In any case, they've become invested in doing one thing really well, and doing it for long periods of time.

Now, imagine what that client's *body* is going through. More specifically, imagine the inputs that it's receiving. That upper back is thinking, "I've got to be hunched like this. This is my new reality. Maybe my human is trapped under a collapsed building, or they're having to roll a boulder up a hill for eternity. I guess I'd better make the best of it." So that upper back gets really good at being *bent* while being *strong*. If you've ever touched an upper back that felt like it was made of hammered rebar, you've met this specimen.

The central nervous system, of course, has its own opinion. While your upper back is doing its best to configure itself for your lifestyle, your brain and spinal cord might see this as a catastrophe. It sees those strained, tense rhomboids as endangered, and it gives you pain as a warning sign. It might even cause spasm to prevent any further harm. That human, broken yet whole, comes to you.

What can you do if you can't fix? You can inform. You can educate. You can do all of this without saying a word.

Think of that beleaguered upper back and imagine what it must be thinking when it gets a massage. "Oh hey, my thoracic vertebrae are extended again. My scapulae are retracted, and there seems to be something rhythmically compressing my muscles in a soothing way. Maybe... maybe I don't need to be bent all the time. Maybe the world's not a terrible place."

How about that central nervous system? "Huh, that emergency situation in the thoracic region seems to have calmed down. We're also getting some powerful analgesic stimuli, along with some psychosocial indicators of safety. Maybe we don't need that pain or spasm right now."

Now, imagine that whole human. They're not just their upper back, or their unconscious nervous impulses. They're all that, plus a history, and a mind, and needs and dreams and fears. They've lived with their hunched back and their pain for a long time, and suddenly they can stand up a little straighter. They can breathe more easily. Not because you've fixed them, but because their parts have calmed down a bit. That whole person might think, "Hey, I could get used to this. What if I stood up like this more often? What if I made some changes so that I could feel like this all the time?"

By calming that emergency situation and helping them feel comfortable, you've created a space for change. You've helped them get a glimpse of a new homeostasis.

Why you shouldn't be scared of "deep tissue"

To start, let's talk about what deep tissue *isn't*. It isn't pressing really, really hard. It's not fixing someone or reshaping their body. It isn't even necessarily contacting deeper structures of the body.

Deep tissue massage is *profound* massage. It's thorough massage. When I think back to the best "deep tissue massages" of my life, I don't think of the ones that used a lot of pressure, or the ones that tried to smash my muscles into new configurations. I think of these qualities:

- **Thorough, informed contact**. If I'm having shoulder pain, I want every aspect of my scapula to be interacted with, and for my shoulder girdle to be mobilized. I want my arm to be moved, and for my pecs to be approached from a few different angles.
- **Smart pacing**. If an area seems especially relevant to my complaint, I want my massage therapist to slow down and explore. If an area is tight, I might want some vigorous work. If things have been at one pace for long enough, change it up.
- **Sensitivity**. This is a big one. If I'm getting deep tissue massage, I don't want *lots* of pressure, I want the *right* pressure. Too much and I might reflexively tighten up. Not enough and I might feel like the massage therapist didn't hear my concerns.

That's it. If you've got these three ingredients, then you've got a winning deep tissue massage in my book. Notice the ingredients that I didn't list: Treating trigger points. Orthopedic evaluation. Myofascial release. Structural integration.

These are all fine ingredients. So are reflexology and acupressure and craniosacral therapy and cupping. It's possible to use any or all of these tools in an excellent deep tissue massage, and it's possible to use none of them. Some of the most enjoyable work I've ever received has been from untrained friends who were just giving my shoulders or forearms a squeeze, magically finding that perfect pressure and pace.

So don't get psyched out by the things you "should" be doing during deep tissue massage. A teacher might have told you that you *need* to strip out the scalenes to have success with thoracic outlet syndrome; that you *need* to release the hamstrings before you can hope to work on the glutes; that you *need* to dig into those trigger points to make them go away. But the human nervous system doesn't seem to be so picky. It doesn't seem to care about correct order or stripping out this or deactivating that.

It cares about thorough work at a sensible pace. Give it that and big changes will follow. It's great to have all those other tools in your toolbelt, but it may be better to think of them as toys in your toybox. There's a world of possibilities open to you as a massage therapist, and there are many ways of creating that space for change. Explore, find out what each client responds to, and discover what you enjoy doing.

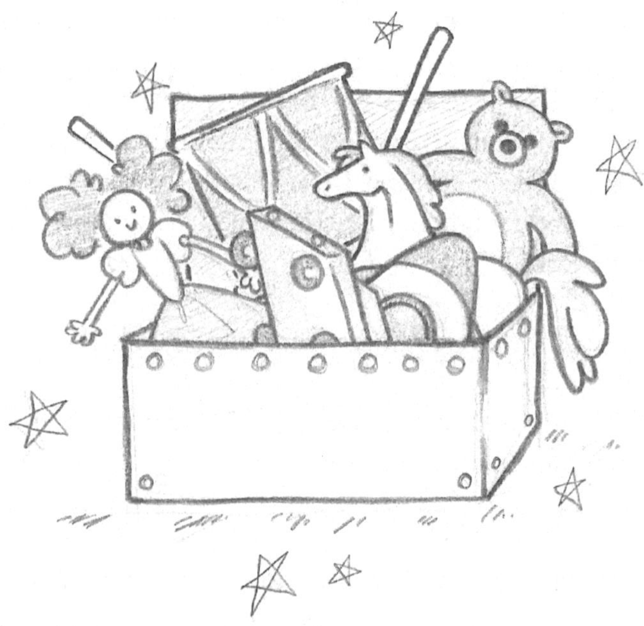

So… we really can't "fix"?

Let me walk that back a bit. The contact that we make has many effects at microscopic and macroscopic scales. As your fist glides along the gastrocnemius muscle, a lot of stuff is happening. Shear forces are being introduced in ways that the body isn't used to, stimulating the nervous system in ways that it doesn't get when the client is just walking around. No matter how gentle you are, the mechanical deformation you create is causing microtrauma in the local collagen and muscle fibers, causing the release of pro- and anti-inflammatory chemical messengers. Fibroblasts and immune cells are getting activated by this chemical cascade and leaping into action.

As you lift a client's scapula and mobilize it, more of that nervous system stimulation and microscopic chaos is happening. You're also causing the subscapular bursae (remember those friction-reducing sacs that the body puts between moving surfaces?) to depressurize and deform in ways they're not used to, which might cause the synovial membranes to secrete more fluid.

As you apply pressure to the thoracic region, the thoracic spine changes shape. Stretch receptors embedded in the fascia send that information to the CNS, letting it know that this new shape is possible. At the same time, the facet joints and intervertebral discs are deforming and decompressing, causing a chemical cascade that may result in collagen remodeling and tissue hydration.

Now, it should be noted that these effects are not unique to massage. These little recalibrations of the internal environment are happening all the time, with every step, with every pushup, with every stretch. A person can change the structure of their body over the course of time just by giving their body function-promoting stimuli. Massage is one such stimulus.

Indeed, these changes will usually be subtle. One workout won't make you stand any straighter, or make your muscles bigger, or relieve your knee pain. 100 workouts, over the course of a year, can make measurable changes in all these areas.

In the same way, a single massage won't break up an adhesion, or soften scar tissue. It won't loosen tight hip rotators permanently or change the lumbar curvature. 100 massages, over the course of a few years, can affect all these things. The scar tissue, via the reconstructive work of its embedded cells, may have softened. The hip muscles may have recognized their ability to stretch, and to live with less tone. The human will have a new awareness of their shoulders and low back, and they may be able to sit at work without turning into a tight ball of pain.

And yes, big changes can happen after a single massage. I've seen many clients get headache relief after a single massage. TMJ dysfunction can resolve after two or three. Wrists stop hurting, frozen shoulders unlock, and sciatica pain drops. How is this possible if we're not changing their structure in big ways? To answer this, we'll need to explore more about how pain works, and why it exists in the first place.

Interlude: How to Deliver Beautiful Deep Tissue

In chapter 2, I tried to take some of the pressure off deep tissue massage. There are lots of ways of creating the "deep" experience, many of which don't require pressing very hard at all.

When I think of deep tissue, here's the stroke I want to deliver as a massage therapist, and the one I love to receive as a client:

- Start with a nice low table, one that allows you to lean your way through your techniques while using straight arms.
- Look at the area of the body in front of you. You might imagine working down the spinal erectors, or up the hamstring into the hip. Notice the unique shape of this client's body, which isn't exactly like any other client you've ever worked with.
- Gently place a hand on that unique shape, allowing it to be a slow and sensitive landing. Let your hand melt onto that surface as you sense the subsurface topography. Is the muscle tissue tight or slack? Can you sense the boney landscape beneath the muscle and fascia?
- Place your other hand, either stacking it on top of your working hand for extra support and easy application of pressure, or placing it nearby. Either way, do so mindfully and carefully.
- With your hands in place, shift your body. Start by allowing your hips or thighs to contact the table, bringing your center of gravity a little over your client. This can be with a powerful lunge stance or a lazy lounge stance. If you've never tried the latter, just imagine giving more of your weight to the table via your hip or thigh, and letting your low back be slack rather than braced. Experiment with both, varying your stance and how strict it is, and remember to play.
- Now, lean toward your endpoint. Allow your upper body to pour its weight into your client via straight arms and loose

shoulders. As you do so, your hands will start to move on their own without you needing to push them.

- As your hands move, continue changing their shape to mold to the client's body. Expand your hands to grab big swaths of fascia, or make them small to carve into nooks and crannies. Doing a bit of both will tell the story of your client's body.
- As your hands proceed, shift your weight so that you continue applying constant pressure. That might mean rotating your hips, or going into a deeper lunge, or taking a gentle step.
- As the technique comes to a good stopping point, you can either change the placement of one hand to begin your next move or remove them both. Either way, do so gradually and mindfully. Removing your hands can be just as meaningful as placing them.

Here's what this should feel like as the therapist: As you shift your body, *gravity* is driving this move. You're just along for the ride. The weight of your body is translated through your straight arms and into your hands. Your hands are changing shape to interface with the landscape under them, driving fascia forward. You'll see the client's body rock and change shape as you travel.

And here's what the client will feel: A force of nature. A crashing wave, or a landslide. Instead of feeling hands pressing or fingers squeezing, they'll feel a confident, constant pressure gliding across and through their body. As their body changes shape, they'll feel the technique to their core, even if there's not a lot of pressure.

By using gravity to do this work, it feels deep. It feels confident and profound, even if there are only five pounds of pressure driving the move. Imagine a shifting tectonic plate, and you'll know what I mean when I say "deep tissue."

Chapter 3: Pain Doesn't Make Sense!

This is one of the areas where I feel like massage students are largely left to their own devices with the hopes that they'll eventually figure things out. In Swedish class we're told that we're soothing painful areas and reducing muscle tone. In neuromuscular therapy (a.k.a. trigger point therapy) class, we're told that pain has a specific origin, that it's usually a distance away, and it can be erased like an errant comma. In structural integration class, pain is all about retraining tight and imbalanced fascia. Sprinkle in some talk of toxins in reflexology class and meridians in shiatsu, and the origin of pain becomes even muddier.

Things seem clearer in anatomy and physiology: Pain is caused by activation of a special type of nerve ending called the nociceptor. Ah, now that's something that makes sense! Now we just need to turn off those nociceptors by... hm, how do we do that part?

Here's where I've got good news and bad news. Let's start with the bad news, as is my preference: It's way more complicated than this, nociception is happening *all the time* and often being ignored by the central nervous system, and the amount of nociceptive stimulus does not directly determine how much pain we experience. In fact, there can be substantial, life-ruining amounts of pain in areas of the body where there is no damage, and where there is no noxious stimulus at all!

The good news: Everything that you learned about relieving pain in massage school is useful, and some of it is even true. Swedish massage *does* offer a soothing stimulus that can drown out the perception of pain, or reduce it by convincing the brain to be less sensitive to nociception (see *central sensitization theory*). Working with trigger points can ease distant pain — possibly by distraction, possibly by directly inhibiting pain referral. Structural integration might not actually change the shape of a client's fascia, but the slow methodical work can retrain their nervous system to allow more ease and comfort. Both reflexology and shiatsu are wonderful ways to work on the body that can leave the client feeling like they're walking on sunshine, often with less pain. Even in the absence of detoxification or meridian manipulation, this is worthwhile work.

Okay, that's all great. All sorts of different approaches are effective, massage is awesome, but... how?! How does massage relieve pain? For the rest of this chapter, realize that we're dealing with an evolving understanding of how pain works, one that has changed considerably in my lifetime.

Acute vs. chronic

First, let's all get on the same page: When we're talking about pain relief in a massage setting, we're usually talking about chronic pain. The kind that lingers long after an injury has resolved, or that gradually shows up in the absence of damage. We're talking "bad" knees and "bad" backs, as well as long-term problems like carpal tunnel syndrome, plantar fasciitis, and bigger systemic conditions like fibromyalgia.

Acute pain isn't something that I really try to touch in my massage practice. If someone comes to me with a big throbbing thumb that they just hit with a hammer, would I try to massage that pain away? No, there's way too much inflammation, there might be tissue damage that won't be apparent right away, and making contact is likely to cause pain while doing little to relieve it.

I have this same thought process when clients have just twisted their ankle or "thrown their back out." Their body is currently in a state of high alert, and directly challenging a painful area could easily lead to spasm, or to further inflammation. For these clients, I recommend reasonable first aid like an Ace bandage, an ice pack or heating pad, and rest. If their pain is severe or debilitating, I recommend that they take a trip to an urgent care center or emergency room.

Quick aside: Some exceptions are neck spasm (i.e., a "crick in the neck"), headaches, and heel pain. While these can fall into the acute category, I find that they respond well to myofascial release when applied within the client's pain tolerance. You'll find all sorts of exceptions and paradoxical rules in our line of work. Massage is weird.

So, let's talk about chronic pain and how to relieve it. In fact, let's start with those big flashy "massage miracles" that you might see other therapists talking about in continuing education classes or on internet forums. How do we erase pain in one easy session?!

The power of the nervous system

When massage miracles happen, this is where: In the powerful computing and reality-simulation engine that we call the central nervous system. In fact, the human body is usually *resistant* to change, both positive and negative! When we're hurt, when we work too hard, when we're sick, our bodies do everything possible to roll back these changes and get us back to a reasonable baseline. The same when we start working out or eating right; our bodies smooth out the blips and try to enforce the status quo. In the past I've described this as the *inertia of homeostasis*. The only way to make change is to overcome this inertia through consistent progress that's big enough to not be reeled back by the body's homeostatic mechanisms.

But what about sudden recoveries from injury or pain? What about when a frozen shoulder is suddenly able to move after a massage? From what I can tell, these are usually in the realm of the brain and spinal cord. The structure remains the same, but the brain decides to stop being such a Gloomy Gus and starts seeing things in a new light.

This is a story about *central sensitization* and *top-down processing*. If you don't know about these concepts, a lot of human responses to pain will be somewhat confusing. Why would we evolve to hurt? Why would someone's uninjured back become a daily source of mental and physical anguish, even leading to total disability?

Central sensitization: The total knob

The main reason, as far as I can tell, is that our central nervous system is great at *listening*. Like any good partner, it pricks up its ears when it hears that we're in pain and really immerses itself in our problems. From a neurological perspective, it takes the input from the pain sensors and turns the volume knob waaay up until it hears every little thing.

This is called *central sensitization*, where the brain and spinal cord amplify stimuli that otherwise might be filtered out. This can be useful in dangerous situations:

- Using a joint that has been painful in the past.
- Doing an exercise that has resulted in injury before.
- Stepping between bushes where there might be thorns.
- Walking on, walking on broken glass.

Makes sense, right? If there's a possibility of danger or injury, your central nervous system listens *as hard as it can* to let you know if you've encountered a problem.

But that can be a problem in and of itself. What if your CNS is listening *too hard*? What if it thinks every little movement is a possible source of injury? What if it noticed a twinge during one shoulder movement, and now it's decided that every shoulder movement is dangerous?

Here's where things get dysfunctional, and pain can be difficult to successfully deal with. These are normal inputs coming from the peripheral nervous system, but... they hurt. There is no tissue damage to your shoulder, but raising it laterally feels like the world is ending. There's nothing structurally wrong with your back, but sometimes it spasms so hard that you have to call out from work for a few days. Why?

This can be because of interpretation by the brain and spinal cord, which neuropsychologists call "top-down processing." Your brain has decided that there is some sort of emergency based on a past crisis, maybe even one that you don't remember. Your spine is convinced that a local state of stretch represents an injury, even if you're sure that it's perfectly normal to bend down to tie your shoes.

Basically, the parts that interpret all the input from your body have decided that there's an emergency, and now it's time to convince it otherwise. This is where massage comes in.

Massage as a central nervous system soother

When I have a client in my office who has all sorts of pain and spasm despite a clean bill of health, I'm thinking about their brain and its interpretation of events. Why does it think there's a problem worthy of pervasive pain, even though an MRI didn't see anything interesting? Why is it convinced that the hip is in danger even though the injury was finished healing ten years ago?

By realizing that some or all of this pain is a matter of false interpretation based on past events, it helps me figure out my game plan. This isn't a matter of stripping out scar tissue or remodeling a muscle, it's a matter of convincing their nervous system that things are already okay! I've come up with a term for this approach, and feel free to forget it immediately: *Hypoalgesic contact.*

Hypo- means "less," and *algesia* means "pain." Basically, if I can offer stimulus that is less painful than the nervous system expects, then I can start to convince it that it's wrong about the state of emergency. If I can offer evidence that there is no reason to be on high alert, it will gradually start to cool its jets.

If you're wondering, this is my current theory of massage and physical therapy. I can't prove it, but I suspect that the movement and compression we provide, and the exercises that PTs provide, all represent stimuli that gradually convince the central nervous system to let down its guard. By providing hypoalgesic contact and movement, we're helping the CNS — a scientist if there ever was one — figure out new hypotheses about the body and the world. By doing stuff that *should* hurt but *doesn't* (at least not in the ways that it has in the past), we're giving our clients a reason to turn down that sensitivity knob and emerge from that emergency.

I might be wrong about this, but it's a theory I like. It doesn't require me to hurt anyone or change anyone's body. If you like this theory too, realize that it's something about which reasonable people might disagree.

Okay, but what about massage miracles?!

I'm usually thinking about the "convincing" process above, but sometimes the central nervous system goes much faster than that. Rather than slowly coming around, it jumps to a conclusion. Back pain just stops, sometimes after a decade. A stiff hip decides to give you 30 extra degrees of motion in one session. What gives?

This can conceivably come from two directions: From the top or the bottom. The top-down processing model is what we discussed above; in this case, the client's brain has decided to drop the state of emergency all at once and signal the all-clear. Based on this new interpretation, there's no need for heightened sensitivity, so it just stops. It doesn't happen often, but it's pretty amazing when it does, because it can be a lasting change.

There's also bottom-up processing. While this usually refers to the raw input from our sensory neurons, I'm using the term to talk about the *reflexes* that are informed by these inputs. This is the stuff that goes on behind the scenes, completely outside of our awareness. Our spine gets input from different kinds of receptors embedded in our various tissues (touch, stretch, position, etc.), and then uses its local processing power to make some decisions. Based on its monitoring of any given area, it will decide how tight to keep the local musculature (this is what makes some muscles *hypertonic*), how much stretch to allow (can't touch your toes? It's because the spine says that's how it's supposed to be!), and whether to pass pain signals along to the brain.

The spine is adept at using *feedback loops* to monitor and maintain your peripheral nervous system many times per second; it gets information, sends out motor impulses, gets feedback on those changes, sends out new impulses, on and on, forever and ever, amen.

This is the realm of the small, everyday massage miracles we see: When you soften up a hypertonic muscle; when you feel the "release" in myofascial release; when you get a trigger point to go quiet. These are all a function of interrupting that spinal reflex feedback loop. How do we do that?

Giving the spinal cord something to chew on

If you want to push the nervous system's pause button, give it something new to think about. Any new stimulus will cause a flood of unexpected information to hit the processing centers in the spine, often giving it a reason to temporarily damp down its sensitivity. This can be used for pain-relieving purposes: When the peripheral nervous system receives lots of new touch, movement, and stretch data, it causes the spinal cord to temporarily reduce its sensitivity to pain (see *gate control theory*). This is probably one way that massage gets results.

Want to interrupt a feedback loop that is causing spasm? Send competing input. The least provocative way to do this is by working with the antagonists of the muscles that are in a state of lockdown. Entire massage modalities are built around this theory of *reciprocal inhibition*, the idea that stimulating the opponents of the distressed muscle will cause it to chill out. This can be seen when we stretch a tight hamstring, then ask the client to powerfully contract their quadriceps, then give that hamstring stretch another try (i.e., PNF stretching). Big new range of motion, as if by magic! For more on this approach, try a good sports massage workshop.

Just realize that while there are a lot of dramatic modalities that can cause dramatic reductions in pain or increases in ROM, I still prefer the slow and steady approach. Yes, I could suppress your pain sensitivity in a few minutes by scraping the overlying skin, or that of the relevant antagonists (see IASTM or Gua Sha); I could leave a cup on one of these areas until the nervous system acclimates to the negative pressure, then remove that stimulus. I could strike the antagonistic muscles with a reflex hammer while moving the joint in a semi-random pattern. I once took an entire weekend workshop devoted to exactly this approach, which was presented as a cure-all.

Offering any new stimulus will often temporarily change conditions enough to dampen pain and spasm. It helps if these stimuli are big and flashy and accompanied by a very confident-sounding explanation for how we're "resetting nerves" or "activating your glutes." It especially helps if it hurts!

On painful massage

If we're trying to turn down a sensitivity knob and convince the nervous system to calm down, why do people do painful massage? Why do clients rave about it and ask you to really dig in until they squirm? Because it works!

It just doesn't work for the reason that most massage therapists claim it does, or for as long as they claim it does. They're not "busting up old scar tissue" or permanently lengthening fascia — you'd have more luck trying to lengthen a leather belt by mashing on it with your thumb. Connective tissue is tough, especially scar tissue.

Painful massage works because it is a high-intensity stimulus that competes with other pain. These massage therapists usually aren't directly provoking the same nociceptors that are currently hypersensitive; they're often working with more superficial structures or nearby trigger points. They're stripping nearby fascia and muscle rather than focusing on an inflamed tendon. This competing stimulus dampens the pain reporting at the level of the spinal cord, and the client stands up feeling better.

Alternatively, they *do* attack the pain directly. They press their olecranon process directly into a spasming muscle and ask the client to activate that muscle, telling them to breathe through the pain. This can also work! Here we're leveraging the body's analgesic mechanisms — your body has ways of turning off overwhelming pain, and these sessions can be excruciating. The client often gets up feeling not only better, but like a million bucks! This is thanks to a release of endorphins, which are basically a free hit of homemade morphine that your pituitary gland doles out when it thinks you've suffered enough.

In both cases, the crash afterward can be truly spectacular. A sudden and extreme reduction in muscle tone is often followed by reflexive tightening, which is a precursor to spasm. A loss of pain sensitivity from endorphin release can make the return of that sensitivity all the more unpleasant, once again creating a good environment for things to seize up.

On top of everything else, these painful massages do damage. You can't repeatedly press your elbow into someone's spinal erectors at the very edge of their pain tolerance without damaging the tissue. This is the cause of post-massage soreness, or even flu-like symptoms like fatigue and fever.

Now, some soreness is normal. Any new activity will cause delayed-onset muscle soreness the first time or two, even if it's just a longer walk than usual. Here's what I say to my clients: "You might be a little sore tomorrow, but it should be about the same as after a good workout. If it's any worse than that, let me know and we'll go easier next time." This kind of soreness usually stops happening after one or two sessions because the body is able to successfully acclimate to it.

But if a client feels beat up and tired after every session with a no-pain-no-gain therapist, why do they keep coming back? Why do they ask that you emulate that approach and "dig in until I cry"?

"I know it works because it hurts"

Because it feels like *medicine.* People expect medicine to be bitter, or to have the sting of a needle. They expect it to have all sorts of side effects. If a treatment doesn't have side effects, how do I know it's not a placebo?

It's also theater. Painful massage creates a powerful experience, even if that experience kind of sucks. But boy, what a session! No other massage therapist has ever gotten that deep, or made me want to jump off the table like that! And when I got up, I could move my hip like I was ten years younger. Sure did hurt the next day though...

Realize that, combined, these sources of perceived authenticity can make all other massage seem fake. It can become a frustrating experience for clients who are used to pain: "Why doesn't anyone around here give a *real* massage?" If you've got a pain-seeker on your table and you don't address these concerns, you could spend a full hour doing good work and still get a complaint at the end.

The answer here is communication. A question I like to ask first-time clients is, "what do you like in a good massage?" I also tell them, "As I work, let me know if the pressure is ever too much. If you're ever clenching your teeth or holding your breath, that's too much. I never want you to suffer in silence." Between these two bits of conversation, I'm usually able to identify the pain-seekers. They'll pipe up with, "oh, you don't have to worry about that, I want you to dig in!"

My response sounds something like this: "I'll definitely do deep work, but I get my best results by staying within your pain tolerance rather than pushing past it. I want to work with your nervous system rather than against it. Is that something you'd be willing to try?" This, plus some more communication while the client is on the table (more on that later), makes the massage a collaborative process rather than one where a client has a certain picture in their mind and ends up with their goals unmet.

So, no pain ever?

Nope — like I said before, painful massage works! It can do an end-run around the neurological gatekeeping that's maintaining the current sensitivity/spasm environment. It can be a powerful activator of our built-in analgesic systems, allowing the client to experience reduced pain for a while. These therapeutic effects can be used judiciously to increase function and reduce sensitivity. They can even demonstrate that pain isn't always an emergency, allowing them to reframe little aches and pains as a normal function of healthy tissue.

Or, painful techniques can be used indiscriminately in a way that increases sensitivity and spasm, convincing a whole generation of clients that "massage is supposed to hurt." Many of those same clients are told that it's a "you problem" because of their toxins, or because "we needed to break up those knots." They come away from their first massage not knowing how wonderful it can feel, and that makes me want to scream.

Instead, let's start with a principle borrowed from our colleagues in medicine and psychology: Start with minimally invasive treatments, see how they work, and then move on to more aggressive treatments if need be. In the context of massage, "minimally invasive" means "least likely to cause mental or physical discomfort."

The continuum of massage intensity

To follow this hierarchy, start with what's most comfortable and with what the client enjoys, and then expand from there if there's no change, or if progress stalls. You've still got your big bag of massage tricks and tools at your disposal, but you choose to hold off on the high-intensity techniques at first.

One example that comes to mind is working with psoas as a first-line treatment for low back pain. Psoas work can feel fairly invasive, and it can feel intense even if the work isn't deep. Why not keep that in your back pocket until you see whether that client responds well to a less invasive approach? I find that my clients with low back pain respond well to hip extensor work, often without focusing specifically on the hip flexors at all.

"But Ian! You've got to balance the hip flexors and extensors! If you just work with the extensors, the client will just be in worse pain!" I'm sorry, imaginary strawman I'm arguing with, but I just haven't found that to be true. People come in with low back pain, we do some nice ironing out of the posterior and lateral hips, and over the course of a few sessions they tend to have less pain.

If my first approach seems to cause no change, or if we've hit a plateau and no more improvement seems to be forthcoming, I'll ask for their permission to experiment. "Hey client," I'll say, "I'd like to try working a little more directly with these painful areas in your hips. That will mean sinking in on those points and waiting for a while. It will be a little intense, but it should never just plain hurt. Is that something you'd be willing to try?" After that, I might try working with tensor fasciae latae, and with iliacus. If there's still some lingering pain, I'll talk them through what psoas work is like, and ask their consent to work with their abdomen.

That's the "continuum of massage intensity." Start with low-intensity strategies that have proven useful in the past, then get informed consent to increase that intensity if need be. That might mean experimenting with more intense or painful modalities, or modalities more likely to leave marks on the skin like cupping or IASTM. It might also mean working around potentially emotionally intense areas, like near the pubis, or deep in the axilla.

I find working my way up this continuum to be a much more human-friendly way of applying massage than just jumping straight to maximum intensity. I think you'll find that a lot of clients will respond well to more generalized work without needing to "breathe through" any kind of discomfort.

"But Ian!" Yes, imaginary strawman? "What if I know *exactly* how to treat my client's pain, and it's by pressing my thumb into the base of their skull for a full minute?" Then I ask that you keep that in your back pocket for now. Something that I had to discover multiple times over my first decade in this business was this: *Lots* of approaches work for any given type of pain.

For headaches, some people use ultra-gentle craniosacral work. Some use intense structural integration or neuromuscular therapy. Some use good old Swedish, or myofascial release. The crazy thing is that *all these people get results*, even with stubborn chronic headaches that have lingered for years. The same with back pain and hip pain and heel pain.

I'm not saying that "everything works on everything," I'm saying that sometimes all a nervous system in crisis needs is new stimulus, and some nervous systems will respond to gentle intervention. If that's the case, why jump straight to the painful, bruising, invasive stuff? Why not start by meeting each client anew and defaulting to body-friendly, hypoalgesic contact? If that doesn't work, then you and your client can choose to try something more intense, acting as partners in figuring out the needs of their nervous system.

Quick caveat: Some clients will have gone through this process already and will know what their body responds to. If a client comes to me and says that deep trigger point work is what gets them out of pain, I'll happily do trigger point work in that first session. I'll try to bring them on board with an intense-but-not-painful approach, but I won't insist on starting at the bottom of the hierarchy.

If I had to summarize this chapter in one sentence, it would be, "no two bodies are the same, so let the client lead the way." Take ego out of the equation, start with what feels good, and let the client's nervous system do the work of figuring out how to be pain-free.

Interlude: Explaining Pain to Clients

A potential client bumps into you in a lobby. As you step onto an elevator together, they ask, "so why does my back hurt, anyway?" You have 30 seconds to explain the human experience of chronic pain in all its complexity. What do you do?!

Here's my elevator speech on pain. Yours might not sound the same, but this is my working theory: "Your back hurts because your body is trying to change your activities or your environment. It perceives a problem based on the inputs you're giving it, and pain is how it communicates that to you. When it goes into spasm, it's basically forcing change to happen, all while creating a protective cast made of tense muscles."

The elevator door opens, and you each head to your respective destinations. But, ah! You bump into each other once again on the way down! This time they'd like to know, "well, how can massage help?" The clock resets on your 30 second timer.

Here's what I'd say: "Massage is a new kind of input that's much different than what your body gets on a daily basis. It's a way of telling your nervous system that it's in a safe place, and that your muscles are able to stretch out and be relaxed. Over time, massage can help convince your hypersensitive nervous system that there is no emergency."

There is, of course, a lot of nuance being left out of these elevator speeches, as well as answers that pertain to individuals with unique circumstances. What about fibromyalgia? What about pain with a structural cause, can massage help with that? What does it mean when you press on my hip and I feel it in my shoulder? Yes, that last question is something that a client asked while on my massage table. No, I didn't know the answer.

And you don't need to know all the answers either, nor do you need to always project supreme confidence about matters of the body. I want every massage therapist to be comfortable with saying, "I don't know," and asking questions to delve into the client's personal experience.

Don't know a lot about fibromyalgia? Yes, you can and should take classes and read books, and follow message boards to learn more about people's lived experience with the syndrome. But none of that is a replacement for the incredible resource that you have right in front of you: A client whose fibromyalgia experience is unlike any other. Their sensitivity and flare-ups and fatigue will be uniquely their own, as well as their past experiences with massage. That's your ultimate resource.

The same goes for any client who walks through your doors with a pain condition or structural difference. Yes, it's great to be sitting on a huge trove of knowledge and past client experience, but nothing beats learning from the client in front of you! Even if every client with multiple sclerosis you've ever seen has preferred lighter pressure, the client in front of you might be different.

For every client, ask about their experience of their body, and about massages they've received in the past. What has helped in the past? Has a massage ever made things worse?

Any client with chronic pain will be an expert on that pain, both through their own experiences, and through research that they've done. Simply realize that you've always got the answers right in front of you, and you'll never have test anxiety again.

Chapter 4. I'm Afraid of Butts

Let's talk about butts, and bellies, and feet, and bodies. This might mostly apply to prospective students or new massage therapists, but I have the feeling some veterans out there are pretty nervous about working on certain areas.

I know I was! You see, I've got something called obsessive-compulsive disorder, or OCD. This isn't something I'm shy about, so it might not come as a shock to any reader who has followed me for a while. It's part of who I am, and who I always was.

It started with excessive hand washing when I was a kid, and then progressed into a pervasive concern about germs and cleanliness in general. In other words, just about the worst possible origin story for a massage therapist that I can imagine.

But here I am, darn it! I've been a massage therapist for fifteen years now, and massage has actually been excellent exposure therapy. By immersing myself in the concept of human touch (with all its messiness), I've been able to gradually deal with my anxiety. So, this chapter will be gross, but we'll both feel better afterward. Join me, won't you?

Our mutual microbiota

The first concept to come to terms with is that we humans are completely covered in life. Every square inch of external epithelium has billions of bacteria, with the exact composition varying based on location and environment. Certain bacteria prefer armpits, others like ears. We've got mites hanging out near hair follicles, and yeast in every crease and fold. This is called our *microbiome*, and it's part of being human. Our personal microbe collection crowds out nasty invasive species, and it trains our immune system not to overreact to benign stimuli.

Think of it as a garden that you're always unconsciously tending, feeding, and watering. Whenever you eat, whenever you sweat, and whenever you wash, you're caring for an entire world's worth of life, and it's caring for you in return.

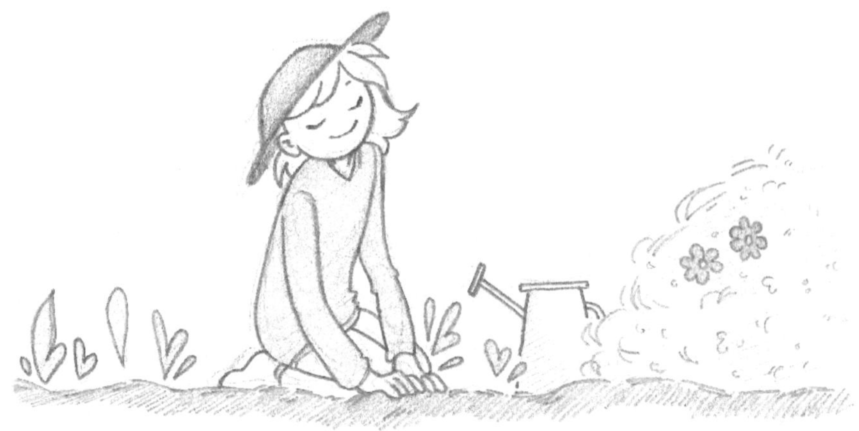

Now, expand that view. No person is an island, and all our personal microbes had to come from somewhere. Indeed, they come from everywhere! Every time you take a seat on the bus or use a machine at the gym or give someone a hug, you're getting a fresh dose of new microbes, and giving them in return! You're also picking up soil bacteria out in nature, and respiratory bacteria during conversations, and fecal bacteria… just about everywhere. Can't be avoided.

And yet, we mostly carry on just fine. In fact, people who interact with dirt more frequently are less likely to have asthma and allergies[4]. Eating fermented foods with bacteria built right in can prevent gastrointestinal distress. Washing too much, especially with harsh chemicals and antibacterial soap, can actually *promote* skin infection by suppressing your friendly neighborhood microbes!

What I'm trying to say is that microscopic life is part of macroscopic life, and we couldn't do without it. We trade bacteria and fungi like Pokémon cards, every hour of every day, and yet we're not constantly beset by infection or illness. Your microbiome is resilient, your skin is strong, and your immune system is a wise gardener.

---

[4] https://www.ncbi.nlm.nih.gov/pmc/articles/PMC2647631/

With some exceptions. Infections do happen. Skin bacteria can go out of whack, as can intestinal bacteria, a problem called *dysbiosis*. Too much of one type of microbe can crowd out others, leading previously friendly bacteria to run amok.

There are also bacteria, viruses, and fungi that love to take advantage of a breakdown in your defenses to quickly multiply or find a new niche. Here we're talking about warts, and herpes, and certain types of candida, among others.

But friends, whether you've got OCD like me and find the thought of talking about this horrifying, or if you've just got a general sense of unease about disease, I've got good news: Catching something from massage is really difficult, because it's simply not an optimal environment for it.

Everything in its place

You see, microbes have environments that they *like*. Foot fungus loves skin folds and nail beds, and it's crazy about prolonged exposure to sweat or other moisture, especially in the presence of broken or irritated skin. A locker room shower is a great place to catch foot fungus due to the conditions above, and due to the sheer number of feet, each one increasing the odds of a successful infection.

Touching a foot on a massage table? Not a great environment for transmission! In fact, the odds are really against the poor candida colony. The environment is fairly dry, and the foot hasn't been stewing in sweaty socks. The hands are usually covered in oil, there's not a lot of friction, and the skin of the hands is intact. How's a fungus supposed to find a foothold in such a situation?

The same with warts, and all manner of skin infections. Like fungus, these are most easily transmitted under a few key conditions: Wet, irritated, and prolonged. On the off chance that you come in contact with herpes gladiatorum (a rare herpetic infection most frequently seen in wrestlers), odds are good that it won't make the successful leap from their skin to your nervous system. It's just not the same as rolling around on a sweaty wrestling mat for a few hours.

And then, there's the ultimate trump card, the defense that's *very* hard for a microbe to work its way around: Handwashing. You'll notice that one of the conditions that allows for transmission is *time*. Fungi need time to multiply before they can overwhelm the local flora. If you deny them that multiplication time by washing them down the drain, you're much less likely to ever know you encountered them in the first place.

The truth is that we're likely to come in contact with all sorts of potential pests as we traverse the integument of 20 different human bodies in a single week. We should, of course, avoid active infections, and keep contraindications in mind. If a client has a lesion or rash they don't recognize, that's a reason to avoid the area until they see a doctor. If there's also a fever or other systemic symptoms, that's a global contraindication, and they won't be getting a massage that day.

But, in general, we don't need to be afraid of the body and its many microbes. Because the conditions are wrong for transmission, and because handwashing is so effective, massage remains a safe way to make people feel more comfortable in their own bodies.

That's… not why I'm worried about butts

Oh, you meant sex stuff! Let's make this a chapter about sex stuff too. Just get all the weirdest stuff in one chapter. That'll be nice.

Massage and intimacy

There's something that we have to lay out on the table before we can have an honest discussion about massage: It's an intimate activity. By that I don't mean "sexual," I mean "up close and personal," often with an element of emotional warmth and a feeling of privacy and safety. It involves contact with usually closely guarded areas of the body, like the feet, buttocks, hamstrings, and ribs, with even the low back having powerful emotional salience for some people.

Sometimes massage therapists see this situation and seem to (consciously or not) rebel against it, making their massage as clinical as possible, or cutting out as many of the normally nurturing aspects of bodywork as they can. I don't want anyone to feel called out here, so I'll call myself out: I was so spooked by intimacy in my first few years of massage that I ended up making my sessions rather unpleasant. I spoke before about seeking and destroying trigger points and focusing on structure. Yes, that was because I found the work compelling, but it was also because it felt *safe* to me. No chance to make anything as awkward as a personal connection if all I'm doing is working on the body like a mechanic! No need for introspection or vulnerability at all!

I was building a wall around myself that made me feel safe in a chaotic environment. I never thought that I was built for spa work, and I only ended up there because they were willing to take a chance on a newly minted massage therapist. Rubbing salt and mud on people? Full half hour sessions on the feet? Couples massages and four-handed massages and hot stones?! It was all overwhelming, and the environment itself was loudly luxurious and pampering, a message blared by soft lighting and soothing music. This didn't feel like "massage therapy" to me. I mocked them for being fluffy and frou frou while employing a badass bodywork ninja like me, secretly on a mission to obliterate pain!

And then I got that complaint. Someone came to a temple of pampering and somehow ended up with an apostate. My manager offered me remedial training with another massage therapist, a chance to shadow her and see how she works. Rather than taking this as a kind gesture and a great opportunity, I took it as another devastating blow to my ego. What can I say, I was a young kid of 26, hotheaded and arrogant.

But after some initial resistance, I took the feedback to heart. I had gone a long way to make my massage practice feel well-armored against emotions that I found scary, and it was time to drop my defenses and evaluate my work. Why did I need my massage to feel so clinical and scalpel-sharp? And would it kill me to light a candle or do some effleurage?

It was around this time that I realized that I wasn't doing a lot of *talking* with my clients. How was I supposed to find out what they needed or expected if I didn't have a little conversation with them? How was I supposed to establish rapport? What was my problem?

The problem was that I was scared. I was scared of intense connections with other people; not just clients, but fellow students and co-workers, and even people passing by in the grocery store. I lived a life of averted eyes and half-mumbled sentences. I was scared of intruding on others' space, or of giving up the little bubble of control I had made for myself. I was afraid of being depended upon, and of needing help. I was terrified of being vulnerable, so I found a small invulnerable way to live.

I wish I could say that I had an epiphany and was able to suddenly explode out of my shell and start living life, but no, that was a process of years (and indeed, it's still ongoing). But with the realizations I made above, I was able to start gradually and gently pressing against my fears. I started with things I remembered from massage school, like doing a more thorough pre-massage interview. It was awkward the first few hundred times, and I said "um" a lot, but I was able to start plotting out more effective sessions. I got back to working with the whole body, and asking for consent if I wanted to leave anything out. I started working with feet every session, even the ones that looked dirty and that triggered my OCD! A cleansing hot towel for them and some hand sanitizer for me was enough to keep my brain from getting stuck in a loop.

I even started lighting a candle. In an essential oil diffuser! I know, groundbreaking stuff.

And in the end, interfacing with intimacy was vital to becoming a better massage therapist. I wasn't doing my clients any favors by focusing solely on pain while ignoring their existence as a whole person. Heck, I wasn't even doing their pain any favors; it turns out that the brain is connected to the body. By embracing the intimate parts of massage, I was able to make the connections that are vital to the therapeutic relationship, and I was able to start having the hard conversations that are so important to finding *just the right pressure* in *just the right place*. It also allowed me to play and experiment, because that's just not possible without real connection and real communication, all within a safe place born of trust.

When intimacy gets confused

Many of us live in fairly low-touch or no-touch cultures. This is one reason why massage can seem like an oasis in a desert – suddenly there's a safe place to receive the contact you've been craving, administered by someone who knows bodies better than anybody. For someone who hasn't felt more than a handshake or hug in years, massage can feel like freedom. It can feel like acceptance.

It can also feel like sex. For a repressed person (and most of us repress our needs and desires to some extent, just to function in the society we're born into), undressing, lying down, and receiving touch can be a powerful reminder of the last time they were in a situation with similar parameters, and it can light up the exact same areas of the brain. Unless this person has been a regular recipient of backrubs and shoulder squeezes from their friends and family, a world I'd dearly love to help build, then they've got few experiences to compare massage to otherwise.

For people like me, this leads to suppression of those alarming thoughts and emotions, shoving unbidden thoughts of sex and intimacy as far into the back of my brain as I can. This can actually be an adaptive and prosocial form of repression: This isn't a sexual circumstance, so containing and damping down those thoughts allows me to enjoy what's really happening, and to feel the input I'm receiving through my touch receptors instead of reinterpreting them as something titillating. After a couple of sessions of experiencing massage as it is, I was able to divide it from sex and appreciate it as a distinct experience.

You'll also encounter people who are able to enjoy massage without pushing away the feelings of intimacy, seeking it for that very quality. These can be people who have felt unsafe receiving touch in the past, whether it be from abuse or internalized shame. These can also be remarkably self-possessed people who realize that intimacy is a vital nutrient in their social or spiritual upkeep, and so they make sure to keep that resource topped up. This is one reason I'm glad that I'm no longer so outcome-focused or pain-centered — I'm able to meet these people where they're at and create the session that helps them feel safe and self-actualized, often with plain old Swedish and no particular focus.

And then, there are the repressed people who translate safety and intimacy directly into sex. Rather than following the social cues that indicate they should suppress that impulse, their misdirected libido leads them to ask, "what if...?" This is often confusing for them, as sex has often been confusing for them, and so you'll get mixed and contradictory signals from these clients, frequently culminating in a clumsy come-on or other inappropriate behavior.

For the clumsy and confused, realize that a brief and clinical response will usually suffice: "I don't do anything sexual here, I just offer therapeutic massage. Does that work for you?" I've had a number of clients make a pass at me, receive a simple "no," and proceed to be model citizens. If they can't leave well enough alone, or if their sexual remarks or requests are beyond the pale, you can send them on their way: "I'm ending the massage here. Please get dressed and meet me in the hall."

There are also predators. This group is not confused at all; indeed, pushing boundaries is something of a hobby for them. I don't want to make this group seem too spooky, because they are few in number and usually bumbling and ineffectual, but I'd be remiss if I didn't give them a thorough accounting.

A taxonomy of creepers

Please note that the following section might be anxiety-provoking for people who have experienced abuse, so feel free to skip it for now, or review it with the help of a trusted friend or counselor.

No matter your gender or age, you're likely to come across someone with bad intentions during your career as a massage therapist. Depending on where you work and how clients find you, you may encounter more or less. I want to make sure that I lead with this: Most clients will be lovely; they'll be there because they love massage or have found it to be powerful, and some will seek you out specifically because they've heard such good things. This will be your day-to-day experience, and once you're busy enough, you may never encounter a single person with bad intentions.

But occasionally, you'll come across someone who seems to be fishing for something, or asking questions that make no sense, or trying to push your professional boundaries. These will almost invariably be men, so I hope you'll excuse me for using the male pronoun here. I also hesitate to call them "clients," because they're not seeking treatment in good faith. For now, let's go with "creepers." I've been cataloguing these types over my career, as well as swapping notes with other massage therapists, so here's a brief field guide:

The Fisherman: This can be the easiest type of creeper to deal with, because they reveal themselves right from the outset. They always start with fishing expeditions, usually in the form of strange questions that *sound* vaguely massage-related, but that are maddeningly weird. Here are some examples:

- "Do you do full body massage?" or "Do you work with every area of the body?"
- "Are you okay working with an older man?"
- "Do you have any hang-ups about the body?"

They'll also volunteer information that most people wouldn't find necessary when reaching out to a healthcare practitioner:

- "I've got a lot of muscle mass, is that something you can work with?"
- "I've got a lot of piercings/hair/tattoos, I hope that won't be a problem."
- "I've got scars [here, here, and here], can you take a look and see if you can help with those?"

Like I said, all the above are vaguely massage-related, and may even be topics that come up with a client in pain. But Fishermen lead with these questions to probe your responses, and to see if you're willing to put up with someone steering the conversation. Watch for strangely aggressive cold calls/texts from unknown numbers who haven't been referred. If they immediately jump to talking about needing work with their inner thighs or glutes (again, normal massage stuff, just in a weird context!), then that pretty much seals the deal.

Try not to let these people bowl you over, and listen to that voice inside that asks, "why are they focusing on such strange things? Why would they need to ask about this?" Once you recognize a fishing expedition, you can say, "I don't think I'll be able to help. Thanks for calling, and have a nice day!" They're used to it, and most of them will move on to the next number on their list.

The Escalator: This type is a little more subtle than the Fisherman, especially at first. While they might throw up some yellow flags during the interview process, they get their kicks from gradually making things more and more explicitly sexual.

They do this by shifting the window of what's acceptable during a session, sometimes taking many weeks to become blatant enough to throw up a clear red flag. They'll often start with boundary-pushing conversation topics:

- "Do guys ever get excited while they're on the table? How do you deal with that?"
- "Do you give your boyfriend/girlfriend massage all the time? They're so lucky."
- "Can you work a little farther onto my inner thigh? No pressure though! I know that makes some people uncomfortable."

Broaching vaguely sexual or personal topics, talking about parts of the body that can be titillating, and asking you to push your own boundaries regarding contact are all fairly typical ploys. They might even play bashful and embarrassed about it, or apologize "if I made you uncomfortable." These are tactics they've found useful in the past to both prolong the boundary-pushing conversation, and to subtly pressure you into pushing past your own boundaries. If they can get you saying, "no, it's okay! I'm not embarrassed," then they've successfully gotten you to dip a toe into the new normal that they're trying to create.

Those in the audience who are familiar with the tactics of abusers will recognize this as *grooming*. Grooming is a form of manipulation where you take a person outside of their comfort zone in a way that is framed as a normal part of conversation or friendship. Getting the recipient of the abuse to apologize for being uncomfortable, or to have them view pressing through the discomfort as an act of courage or maturity, are seen as victories for the groomer. Anything to get the recipient off balance and feeling like the shift is their own idea.

Eventually, the Escalator will find ways of testing the results of their boundary pushing. Talking about the sex they had the night before, shifting the drape to expose more skin, or to emphasize their genitals (which they might "apologize" for). Making more contact with you before, during, or after the massage. He might also engage in subtly sexual behavior on the table, like "adjusting himself" more than is strictly necessary (once after a flip is normal, ten times isn't), or shifting his hips on the table while face down.

Some of these will seem almost normal by this point: "That's just how he is" or "that's just how we are." Even the possible self-stimulation will seem subtle enough that you'll be left asking, "was he doing something wrong, or am I imagining things?" By pushing boundaries more and more while acting like things are normal, this becomes a form of *gaslighting*. Gaslighting is a type of manipulation where the abuser uses subtle or overt forms of reality denial to make you feel like you're being irrational when you're just trusting your own eyes or memory, or like you're the aggressor in a situation where you're being harmed. It can leave you feeling unbalanced and indecisive, and even like you've done something wrong.

When he finally does something that completely crosses the line, such as exposing himself or masturbating under the sheet, it can *sometimes* feel possible to finally eject him, or at least send an email telling him not to come back. Or, it can feel like the therapist has allowed so much, or let the relationship become so sexual, that it was all their fault and that they failed as a professional. It can even feel like it's easier to simply let it keep happening, because things have already gone so far. The massage therapist might feel scared to speak up, or to ask for help, because they feel ashamed, and even complicit.

It happened to me, and I'll tell you what I was able to eventually tell myself: It wasn't your fault, and you have nothing to be ashamed of. You got rudely used by someone who has done such things before, and it has nothing to do with your professionalism, or what energy you put out, or how nice you were.

My friends, we don't have to coddle abusers, either in person or in our memories. We don't have to say, "yeah, but I let him get that far." Yes, you can use this as an opportunity to shore up your defenses and figure out future contingency plans, but no, you weren't the one who did wrong. These guys know what they're doing, even the ones who play dumb as part of their act.

How to prevent this? Keep an eye out for those initial attempts at escalation and respond by being brief and blunt, by being as drily clinical as possible, or by being silent. If they ask, "So, do guys ever get excited on the table? Is that awkward?" you can respond with, "I'd prefer not to talk about that." It can be scary to be that blunt the first few times, but manipulators count on people not wanting to be seen as rude, even while they themselves are being exceptionally rude. This also works for discussions about politics and religion, by the way.

If they say, "can you work farther up onto my inner thigh? Sorry if that seems weird," you can say, "that's not an area I work with," or "the hip adductors aren't something that I directly address." And no, it doesn't matter if these answers are true. If you're getting the feeling that this person is trying to search for weaknesses in your defenses, it's time to drop a brick wall in front of them.

What if you're wrong and this person was just trying to be friendly? Then they'll stop probing and start just enjoying their massage. What if they keep pressing? Then it's time to drop them! I'll talk more about that in the next section. For now though, let's meet:

The Naked Man: This is the most startling creeper of all, because he's just so darn brazen. Here's how it usually goes: You have a lovely intake with a delightful man (sometimes older and rather fatherly), you're able to discuss his treatment goals and talk about areas of his body that might be relevant to his pain. You give your carefully crafted speech on how much to undress and how to lie on the table. You leave, wait, knock on the door, and BAM, you're greeted by the sight of a naked dude, face-down on top of the drape, butt and bits exposed to the elements.

At this point, it's normal to wonder whether there has been a miscommunication. He must have misheard that part about being under the drape, even though you lifted the drape a little and pointed under them! Yes, just a mistake, and I bet he's just as embarrassed as you are. You might be tempted to say, "Oh! Sorry! Under the top sheet please!" before closing the door again and waiting out in the hallway. At this point he might yell an apology, or something like, "it's okay, I don't mind!"

Yes, you might be able to wrangle this person into acting right for now, but I guarantee that he'll try something again, or push your boundaries in less brazen ways. So, my recommendation is this: If you walk in and see an obvious red flag, act on it. If you work in a group environment, have your front desk staff or a colleague escort them out. If it's just you, have yourself a nice yelled conversation through the door: "Mr. Johnson, I need you to put your clothes back on and meet me out in the hallway. That's right, please dress and collect your personal items, I'll see you out here." If you feel at all unsafe, then exit the establishment yourself rather than meeting them in the hall. Your personal safety is more important than your office or your stuff. Give their phone a call and ask them to please leave and not come back. Calling the police is also a fine way to deal with someone exposing themselves, especially if you feel at all threatened.

It won't always be the bare bottom that they start with. This same type of fellow might also simply pull the top drape to the side, perhaps talking about being too hot. Yes, you can offer them a fan or to turn the air down, but you don't have to indulge their paper-thin ploys. A Naked Man might also place his hand on your body as you pass, or start stimulating himself, or ask for sexual services out of the blue.

This can be shocking, but it can also seem surreal, especially because they'll usually do it in the same charming demeanor that they had during the intake. These men often make a point of talking about their wife and kids, building up their credentials as totally-not-a-creep. Give yourself points if you recognize this for what it is: Gaslighting. They're using an aura of normalcy to try to trick you into thinking that you're imagining things, or that their behavior is somehow acceptable. "He must not have been masturbating, he was chatting amiably about his lunch date with his wife!"

How do you kick someone out who's being a perfect gentleman, all except for the suspicious movement of hands or hips under the sheets? You don't need to confront them or accuse them (though you can!), you can just use "I language." "Mr. Johnson, I feel uncomfortable and I'm going to end the session. I'm going to leave the room, please get dressed and meet me in the hallway." This is also the language that you can use in an email or text after the session: "I felt uncomfortable and am cancelling all future sessions. Thank you for understanding." By using language focused on your experience rather than saying, "you were doing this," it makes it much harder for them to argue or engage in further gaslighting. If they try anyway, just repeat yourself and wait for them to get the picture and go away. I doubt it will be the first time they've been booted, and most predators retreat at the first sign of resistance.

Creeper-proofing your practice

I know that reading about the jerks and abusers who can find their way onto a massage table can be scary, and it can even make you wonder why you'd want to go into a field where people think you can be mistreated. It's normal to be frustrated that these people exist, and to be wary of them. I just ask that you remember this: Most clients, the vast majority, are there to experience massage for what it is and for how it can enhance their wellbeing. They're looking for that oasis in a desert of touch-deprivation and cookie cutter pain treatment, hoping for someone to finally connect with their frazzled nervous system. As a massage therapist, you will see amazing recoveries from pain and dysfunction that had seemed impossible, and you'll make long-term connections with clients who see your practice as a vital way to manage stress.

In the end, those occasional encounters with guys with bad intentions will seem like no more than a rare blip in a field of fulfilling therapeutic relationships. That said, it'd be nice to be able to reduce the frequency of those run-ins, and to nip them in the bud if they do manage to get through. How do you ward against them?

1. **Fill your books to bursting**. Creeps are, by and large, very bad at dealing with delayed gratification. They want to be gross, and they want it now. So, if your schedule is full to the brim with regular clients and your next available appointment isn't for two weeks, the *vast* majority of bad dudes will look elsewhere. It's also a simple numbers game: If your book is full of clients you love, the potential for mayhem of any sort goes down. It's a great way to have a predictable schedule, a predictable income, and a mellow and enjoyable work life.
2. **Follow your instincts**. When you sense those warning signs, blow an old-timey coach's whistle in your head and call a timeout. Abusers of all stripes thrive in environments where people feel the need to be polite or deferential, and it's how they find cracks in people's boundaries that they can exploit. They deal *very* poorly with brick walls, so drop one of those when you first get that gut feeling. If a guy seems to be fishing with weird questions, ask him, "what makes you ask that? I'm trying to figure out the purpose of your question." Sometimes this is enough to separate the creepers from the awkward clients. If they continue showing warning signs, you can simply tell them, "I won't be able to take you on as a client, thank you for calling and have a nice day."
3. **Manage how people find you**. Casting a wide net can be a fine way to find lots of clients, but it is also chaotic. If you run a Groupon campaign, you will get a mix of bargain shopping tourists, bargain *snobs* (only the highest standards for their $20 services!), nice folks who are interested in trying different

massage therapists (some of whom will be a great fit), and creeps. If you run a Facebook or Google ad campaign and target it at every person within 10 miles of you, you'll get a similar motley mix of good fits and misfits. Focus your ad money on demographics that represent your favorite clients to work with (e.g., nurses, athletes, office workers, or whoever sparks your therapeutic instincts), and then let word of mouth do its work. See Chapter 7 for more on client outreach.

4. **Practice your professional power**. If a creeper does creep through, a really good feeling is being able to stop him in his tracks, shoo him out the door, and get on with your day. This might sound difficult, but it's only hard the first time, and... it can be kind of fun after that. If you're usually fairly timid like me, it can feel good to flex that assertiveness muscle. My recommendation is to practice what you'll say to clients who are acting inappropriately, first in a mirror and then eventually with a trusted colleague or fellow student. Remember the tips from above: Be brief, use language focused on your experience ("I feel uncomfortable"), and offer no apology or other explanation.

If you ask about how to deal with creepers on message boards, you'll often get advice about how you're presenting yourself, or the language you use, or how you should come across as more clinical and severe. Basically, wear scrubs, don't smile, and don't have a personality. But screw that, and screw the patriarchy. Creepers don't creep because of how you look or what you say, they do it because they've got some deep-seated psychosexual pathology that morphed into antisocial behavior over time. I've never met a massage therapist who works in a spa or franchise setting who hasn't dealt with a creep or five, and the frequency didn't correlate at all with how the therapist looked or dressed.

Be yourself, boldly and without apology. Allow yourself to be vulnerable and invite the same from your clients, all within the safe sanctum of the therapeutic space you co-create. And when someone throws up a warning sign or makes your spidey sense tingle? Catapult them into the sun, take some time to process, and then keep being yourself. We can't let bad actors define us, and this is a problem that can be mitigated. And, because most clients are lovely and there for *you* and the experience you offer, eventually these oafish outliers will be crowded out completely and will be remembered as brief and rare blips.

So uh… what if I'm still scared of butts?

In this chapter we talked about germs and why you don't need to worry about them too much. I feel like that went pretty well. We also talked about how massage is inherently intimate and how that can call to confused or ill-intentioned dudes. I tried to be reassuring during all of that, but is it really worth working with butts and feet and bellies if it's just going to give people the wrong idea? Wouldn't it be better to just leave those areas covered and not touch them at all?

I say no. In fact, I'd like to say, in the strongest terms I'm capable of: Heck no.

I've got two reasons for this. First, we can't allow ourselves to be defined by what might happen if our intentions are misconstrued. That can lead to gradually contracting our forms of expression, compressing ourselves into a tiny safe box, until no one can ever hurt us. When I was younger that meant never looking anyone in the eye and never speaking up. In massage that might mean mostly working with the back, and never passing inferior to a strict line around the fifth lumbar vertebra. It might mean being brisk and clinical in every communication so that no one can think you're a valid target for sexual desire.

But this is a trap. It's a trap because no amount of strictness or medical ornamentation will be enough to ward off a determined creep — it's not about who you are, it's about who they are. You can't make yourself invincible in a chaotic world, so make what changes you can, and otherwise be prepared to nip bad behavior in the bud.

My second reason for not just leaving those potentially awkward areas covered: Because they're *awesome*. I love gluteal work. I love abdominal work. Both giving and receiving. These areas are so rarely touched, and *so full of potential.* People are walking around half-hobbled by the ravages of their 50-hours-a-week desk jobs, with underpaying bosses literally changing the shape of their employees' bodies just so that they can adapt to some ungodly office chair. Their shoulders and wrists hurt, yes, but their butts are crying out for a way to decompress.

This frequently gets translated into low back pain. When you get a client in your office with low back pain, make sure to have them point out on their bodies where the pain is felt. Some will point to their lumbar region, but many will point directly to the sacroiliac joints! There might be some element of pain referral, but I think it's mostly that people are so out of touch with their own pelvis that they can't recognize when it's the epicenter of pain and spasm. The same with shooting pain down the leg; make sure to specifically ask about gluteal pain or numbness, because people often don't think to mention it, or they feel like they're not allowed to.

My first massage ever was at a chiropractor's office. I was there for my chronic and persistent low back pain, and... the back cracking hadn't really been helping, but hope springs eternal. One day they offered me a massage slot that happened to be open, and the massage therapist did some excellent compressive work on my glutes through my boxer briefs. I could *feel* the connection between that compression and my pain, and suddenly my eyes were open to a vital truth about my body: I needed to start thinking about my hips!

In fact, I had allowed myself to become completely alienated from that part of my body, and I barely knew it existed. I think that's something that happens to a lot of people, especially people with chronic pain. They start thinking of a knee as a "bad knee," and suddenly it's no longer invited to the body's family reunions or group chats. Pain warps how we relate to ourselves, and it can result in people going through life rather disembodied, feeling like a mech pilot up in the head rather than a whole person.

And for people like that, massage can be a revelation. Even without "fixing" or otherwise making changes, massage can bring the body together in a way that the client hasn't felt since they were a kid. Suddenly they're able to see how the leg bone is connected to the hip bone (etc., etc.), all in a soothing way administered by an expert who projects an aura of acceptance and support.

Okay, butts are scary

There, I admitted it. At least, they are to me. Buttocks can carry sexual connotations, they're near neighbors to excretory and reproductive orifices, and for a lot of people, they can feel quite private, and even anxiety-provoking. I want to work with butts (and bellies, and feet) because there's so much potential for pain reduction and self-reunion; I want to work inclusively because the body is all connected and inextricable from the nervous system. Your body is you, and you are your body, and I'm here to work with a person, not a part.

How to navigate this emotionally fraught world of the body? With thorough communication and a set of best practices at hand.

1. Acknowledge the intimacy. It might feel truer to say, "acknowledge the awkwardness." Consider this for both parties: You might be feeling awkward about asking to work with the hip rotators, and they might find the thought a little scary. Keep this in mind, and keep in mind how you used to feel before you conquered your fears. Remember what it was like to be a first-time massage client. A beginner's mindset will always serve you well.
2. Open the floodgates of communication. Before you start talking about how you'd like to approach their pain, start with a thorough interview, one in which you give them plenty of time and space to start talking. Ask open-ended questions and let them ramble. When they're on the table, keep giving them opportunities to speak up.
3. Seek informed consent. If that phrase has stopped having meaning to you because you hear it so often, informed consent has three necessary parts: Information about *why* you'd like to proceed a certain way and *what* you plan to do; a request

for consent to proceed; and explicit encouragement to rescind that permission at any time if they feel the need.

4. Before you work with potentially emotional areas of the body, communicate. As you work with that area, communicate. Give your client plenty of chances to speak up, to talk about their experience, and to have you back off if need be.
5. Let safety be a powerful and pervasive force in your massage room and in your work. Frequently anchor the drape to the upper sacrum using a broad, reassuring hand as you work with the exposed hip. Prevent drafts and drape slippage by crumpling fabric and tucking in non-threatening areas (I find tucking the drape just above the knee to feel much less intimidating than a more proximal tuck, for instance). Remember the direction of your fingers as you travel so that clients are never worried about where you're headed next. Put yourself in their shoes and anticipate what will feel safe and reassuring.
6. Never take permission for granted after receiving it once, especially across sessions. While a client might be happy to receive anterior neck work one session, they might feel a little wary about it on the day they got yelled at by their boss or shoved on the subway. Your client's body is always their own.

Let's say a new client comes into my massage office with low back pain and numbness in their left posterior thigh. In my clinical opinion, *something* is going on with their left-side hip muscles, likely interacting with their sciatic nerve. I could just tell them, "I'll need to work with your hip" and power through the interview, trying to skip to the part where I can obliterate their pain! But that would suck, and I would suck if I did that.

Instead, I conduct a nice long interview that eventually homes in on that main area of complaint. I ask open-ended questions about their experience, and the client feels safe enough to volunteer that "sometimes it hurts really bad after I do a plank." Not unusual for there to be a connection there, and that gets me thinking about the hip flexors that are so powerfully activated in that position. I ask about pain along the front of the hip, and yes, there's an ache there that flares up after a long day of sitting. Interesting! Great info! But I'm not ready to get attached to any one hypothesis yet, so I make a note of it in their chart for future investigation and keep the interview moving.

When they talk about their low back pain, I have them show me exactly where they feel it. They point directly to their left SI joint, and then volunteer that it can spread outward from there. I ask about the hamstring numbness and have them point that out, and they volunteer that it can travel all the way to their toes. Great info! Still not getting attached, but I do have a tentative plan, and it serves us both well if I let them know what I'm thinking and why.

"So, this area that you pointed to is your sacroiliac joint, your SI joint, and it attaches the bottom of your spine to your pelvis. A lot of muscles attach near here, all of which control the hip! I suspect that there's some tension in these muscles, and that might also explain that travelling numbness sensation down your leg. There's a big nerve that passes through and near this group of muscles called the sciatic nerve, and it might be getting compressed. I'd like to work directly with these muscles, these muscles here, and try to get them to give up some of the tension, is that something you'd be willing to try? Okay great. If I'm ever too far into your personal space, or if you just don't like it, let me know and we'll try something else."

As I explain this, I make sure to point out on my own body exactly where I'm planning to work, so that there's no confusion or surprise. I'll go on to explain about undressing and undraping, once again letting informed consent and a feeling of safety be my guiding lights.

Creating a refuge

It's in this environment that trust can be forged. It's a place where protective walls can be let down. I've talked a lot about what pain is already, but here's something else pain can be: Pain can be fear, and tight muscles can act as another protective wall. Pain is something the body uses to keep us safe, so it makes sense for people who live with constant fear or anxiety to have an exaggerated pain response. It makes sense for their muscles to create armor to guard them when and where they feel vulnerable.

Once again, the answer here isn't to run away from that vulnerability or to pretend it doesn't exist. It doesn't serve anxious clients to wave away their anxiety and bowl them over with *your* treatment plan. This can be the quickest path to getting them on the table and getting the session started, but think of how much could be accomplished by meeting them in that vulnerable place and discussing their fear and their pain. You can learn about exactly where they need work and how best to apply it. By meeting them where they are and interfacing with their body in a way that it can comfortably accept, you'll find that you can accomplish amazing things together.

Imagine a client who has had shoulder surgery with a poor outcome, and who has since stopped using that shoulder for much of anything. It hurts, physical therapy hurts, and everyone who has ever worked with it just caused more pain. Instead of going down the path of trying to "fix" that shoulder or force it to act differently, you talk to that client about their pain. You see the worry on their face, and you ask, "this has been a big problem for you, hasn't it?" The client admits that they feel like their life has changed completely, dividing their story into before-surgery and after-surgery. Their sleep is terrible, it's hard to put a shirt on, and every medical professional they see either causes them pain or dismisses them. How can you work with an area that's burdened with so much fear and alienation?

Start with communication and consent. "Jane, I'd like to work with this area, but I'd like to try to do so in a pain-free, comfortable way. It will be very slow, and it might not feel like I'm doing much at all, but I'm hoping we can gradually get the surrounding muscles to ease up a bit. Is that something you'd be willing to try?" Over the course of several sessions, you envelop that shoulder in kind, nurturing touch. Rather than trying to fix or force, you interface with the nervous system and what it can safely accept that day. Over time, you and Jane find that you can guide it into slow, gentle circles as you work, a motion that would have been fairly scary for her previously.

As weeks pass and you continue this conversation with her shoulder, you're able to bring it into partial flexion, and even have her engage in some active movements.

At this point, for the first time in months, she's having an easier time putting on shirts, and her sleep isn't so terrible. You're able to encourage her to start using that shoulder in her personal life more frequently, and she gives it a try. Within another month or two, she's back to having two shoulders, neither of them "bad."

Embracing vulnerability without expectation

Whether you're working with butts or bellies or surgical sites, realize that you're always working with a whole person. I strongly believe that our best results come from a meeting of the minds rather than any technique or modality. If you're working with suspected sciatica, the whole process will work better if it's done in a way that feels safe, using pressure and techniques that honor the pain and tightness in the area. Start with what the nervous system can comfortably accept and expand from there as it allows.

This is going to sound crazy, but you can do this without an agenda. You don't need to think, "this process is only worthwhile if I can eventually work directly with his psoas." You're not melting down defenses so that you can get to "the real work." Creating a safe place and using person-centered massage *is* the real work. Every session is worthwhile, even the ones where the client is tentative about receiving touch and remains stiff as a board.

This is all part of a process of self-acceptance and partnership. Allow that process to lead wherever it leads – for some people, it will lead to freedom from pain. Some people who seemed to be made of iron will eventually allow themselves to sink into the table and let you pluck their shoulder blade up and mobilize it. Some people who had self-stigma about their belly or their "gross feet" or their "back fat" will be able to set those ideas aside as they step into the sanctuary you've created together.

And some people will seem the same after session twenty as they seemed after session one. No progress with their muscles, no real connection! They still keep their boxer briefs on, even though you know they'd benefit from direct hip work!

I want you to embrace that too. Accept that person, realizing that your concept of rapport or a strong therapeutic relationship might not map the same way onto every client. I've talked about the value of working with infrequently contacted areas and how that can lead to pain relief and body-integration, but I encourage you to leave that as a value that you hold rather than a goal that you pursue.

It's rewarding when progress is visible and a connection is forged, but for some clients, the benefits they receive from massage will be completely behind the scenes. There are no miracles or revelations, and that client's back still feels like a brick wall. And yet... they continue coming back, week after week. You ask how they felt after their last session, and they say, "fine." Can that be enough?

If you ask me, that sounds pretty great. They've found their massage therapist, they're getting work that makes them feel good, and by all appearances, they're content. No miracles. No revelations. Just simple satisfaction.

As I ask you to consider your own vulnerability and the weirdness and intimacy of massage, what I want most of all is for you to find satisfaction as well. Neither fear intimate connections, nor chase them. Neither fear failure, nor chase success. Allow yourself to be who you are as a massage therapist, meet each client where they are, and create a safe and nurturing space. That is the fertile soil in which a satisfying practice can grow.

Interlude: Considering Trauma

Content warning: This section contains a discussion of trauma, abuse, and post-traumatic stress disorder. If these concepts are anxiety-provoking for you, consider reading this part with a trusted friend or counselor.

As we talk about working with sensitive areas and meeting people where they are, I'd be remiss if I didn't mention trauma and the ways it can impact chronic pain and the ability to receive touch.

Many clients, quite likely most clients, have experienced traumatic episodes over the course of their lives. Violence, sexual abuse, emotional abuse, episodes of profound powerlessness and loss. Any or all of these can lead to lasting emotional and physical effects. When these are severe enough to interfere with everyday life, we call it *post-traumatic stress disorder* (PTSD).

Common symptoms of PTSD[5] are:

- **Hypervigilance and physical guarding**: Remaining on high alert much of the time, with the sympathetic nervous system firing on all cylinders. This can be expressed as tight muscles and difficulty "allowing your arm to be loose."
- **Fatigue and sleep disorders**: Sleep can be disrupted, often by nightmares, with the sleep disruptions exacerbating other symptoms.
- **Emotional suppression**: Keeping their emotions strongly in check, or being unable to connect with their own emotional state. This can result in *flat affect*, which might look like disinterest or dissatisfaction. A good reason not to judge the outcome of your massage by how you *think* your client is feeling.
- **Flashbacks and dissociation**: Reliving a traumatic event or otherwise losing touch with their current surroundings.

---

5 https://www.ncbi.nlm.nih.gov/books/NBK207191/

These episodes are usually rare and self-limiting in nature. They require no intervention on your part, other than to make sure your client is secure on the table and is helped to feel safe after the disturbing event.

- **Irritability, depression, and/or mood swings**: This can make a client seem snappish or withdrawn, and they might be prone to rapidly changing moods.

Realize that people with PTSD can have widely varying presentations of symptoms, and no two will be alike. Hypervigilance and depression are very common, but the other symptoms can be present or absent, or have an atypical presentation. In other words, don't try to anticipate the internal world of someone who has undergone trauma; instead, allow yourself to fully see the person in front of you.

Let's say that you learn that a client is living with PTSD. They feel safe enough with you to share this fact, or they've found that getting it out in the open can be useful when dealing with medical professionals. They might even be in your office specifically to help deal with their PTSD symptoms! How can you alter your session to give this person their best possible massage?

Fortunately, you've got the ultimate resource right in front of you. Ask your client a few questions: What are they looking for in a massage? If they're not a first-time client, what has worked for them in the past? What hasn't worked? You can even say something like, "I'm interested in how your PTSD interacts with massage. Is any part of the process hard for you? Is there any way I can make you more comfortable?" You don't need to know everything about mental health or a particular mental illness in order to ask questions and learn more about the client in front of you. You also don't need to know exactly the right things to say, or the right ways to react. Just be present with your client, and let them lead the way.

PTSD is often associated with chronic pain, and even a paradoxical relationship with pain[6] and muscle tension. A client with

---

[6] https://pubmed.ncbi.nlm.nih.gov/18585862/

PTSD might have broadly distributed pain, from headaches to plantar fasciitis and everything in between, along with joint issues and gastrointestinal distress. They might only have a couple of these issues, or there might be problems that come and go. Again, the client in front of you is the best guide to their own areas of concern, and they can lead the way on how to customize their session.

Some possible customizations you might encounter:

- For some people, not just those with post-traumatic stress, a face cradle can feel too enclosed, or can feel like it's causing breathing problems. For these clients, you can place a big pillow longitudinally under their chest and abdomen, with a smaller pillow under their head, allowing them to turn their head to one side or the other as needed. You can also use side-lying massage to avoid prone positioning altogether.
- You might find that a client with hypervigilance is unable to enjoy the feeling of being stretched, and that it can even be counterproductive as their muscles tighten in response. You might also find that their muscles stay contracted no matter how hard they try to "give you their arm," which can end up feeling like a tug of war. If a client isn't getting anything out of these techniques, consider just leaving them out! You might give it another try in a future session to see if things change, but it's normal for this to be a long-term situation.
- You might need to make your movements more obvious and predictable. If you find your client tensing up every time you place your hand, try making each placement less distinct. Instead, move one hand while the other is still working, as if you were taking little baby steps. Do these overlapping placements in nearby areas so that there is never any surprise about where your hand will go next. You can ask your client if they'd like to be informed of what's going to happen next, which would sound like this: "John, I'm going to uncover your left leg and give it a quick tuck. And now I'm going to place my hands on your ankle." You don't need to narrate your entire

massage, but this can help to fill in the gaps where your next move might seem unpredictable to a prone client.

There are a few potential pitfalls here that I'd like to point out: While it's important to work with areas of pain and tightness, it can lead to accidentally ignoring the whole person. You might find yourself so involved with those tight traps that you never do a long stroke down the whole back! Collaborate with your client to try to find the right balance of specific work and holistic integration (i.e., big, broad, feel-good strokes that communicate safety and acceptance).

Another pitfall would be to attack tight areas too vigorously, trying to physically break down a barrier. These clients might even request extra deep or specific work, as some people with PTSD experience a higher than usual pain threshold (this is that "paradoxical relationship with pain" that I mentioned earlier). When working with tight muscle, remember that hypertonicity is caused by nervous system activity. If the spinal cord says that a muscle should feel like a slab of concrete, it will continue to do so until it's told to do otherwise. So, instead of trying to beat down those walls, have a conversation with the nervous system: Come at the muscle from a lot of angles, with the body in different positions, and see if you can convince the central nervous system to allow the peripheral nervous system to chill out. If your client would prefer deep, painful work, communicate with them and see if you can bring them on board with a less direct approach.

Finally, just because tight muscle and chronic pain can be associated with PTSD, that doesn't mean that it's "all in their head." The same goes for the diffuse body pain that can come with depression, the headaches and migraines that are associated with anxiety, and so on. The brain talks to the body, and the body talks to the brain. In the case of hypervigilance, the brain is keeping the autonomic and somatic nervous systems on high alert. Over time, postural muscles stay in a shortened position, muscles and tendons become irritated, and the body reports a painful, distressed condition to the brain. The two keep each other in a feedback loop that can be pretty miserable, causing pain and dysfunction, and reinforcing the apparent need for hypervigilance.

So, while this problem is perpetuated by the ongoing response to past trauma, it is also a physical phenomenon that we can work with. We can intercede in that feedback loop between body and brain, just by creating a space that feels safe to our client, and by communicating comfort with our hands. As always, don't feel like you need to "fix." You don't need to know the perfect approach, and you're not a failure if the client is still tight and tense after your session. This is a long-term problem, and you can be part of the long-term solution. They've got their mental health professionals, friends, and fellow survivors to help them mentally and spiritually. They've got you (and their own activity regimens, and maybe a personal trainer or yoga instructor) to help them physically. And all of this meets in the middle, in the whole person.

In other words, don't feel like you need to be a mental health expert to work with a client living with PTSD. Your work with their body can help their state of mind, just like their talk therapist can help their body. The same goes for every client: You don't need to be anything other than a massage therapist, even for clients in a lot of pain. Let massage be your medicine, let time do its work, and encourage your clients to pursue many avenues of wellness and recovery.

Living in a world of survivors

While the advice above applies to clients who talk to you about having PTSD, you will inevitably see many other clients who have survived trauma. These episodes might be many years in the past or much more recent; they might have been severe and recurrent or mild and transitory. These clients might have no symptoms of post-traumatic stress whatsoever, or they may display the characteristic symptoms so overtly that you can't help but make an armchair diagnosis in your head.

I ask that you leave those hypotheses aside for now. Are you working with someone who is dealing with the after-effects of trauma? There's no way to know without asking, and that falls outside of our purview as massage therapists. Instead, I'd like you to extend the same grace and kindness to every client, no matter your perception of their guarding behaviors or seeming vulnerability, and even if it means setting your usual methods aside.

If a client has difficulty giving up the tension in their arm, preventing you from doing your favorite mobilization technique, you can try some communication and movement strategies. You can ask them to tense and release, and you can give their arm a little shake. But if that arm remains rigid despite your tried-and-true techniques and your client's best efforts, then work with that arm as it is, not how you'd like it to be. Whether it's a hypervigilance behavior or just the way their nervous system is wired, you can still get a lot of work done without a floppy arm at your disposal.

Does your client leave their boxer briefs on, even after ten sessions? Do they tuck the drape extra tight under their arm to prevent it from shifting, or seem to tense up when their thigh is rocked? You could get frustrated by how this messes with your flow, or you could extend grace to that client and think, "they don't need a reason or an excuse; this is their session and their body, and I'll honor their boundaries."

You can communicate about these issues, which I'm always a big fan of: "Jeff, I'm wondering how to work with these boxer briefs in a way that's comfortable for you. Would you mind if I scoot the fabric up your leg before I work, or would you prefer I keep it right where it is? Would you mind if I work through the fabric so that I can work with your hamstrings and hip, or should I stay out of that area entirely?" These conversations don't need to be done all at once, and you don't need to say them perfectly.

Try this format: "I notice that, and I'm wondering if." This is useful for all manner of potentially awkward or sensitive conversations about the body, and about possibly unconscious client behavior. "I notice that there's some tension as I rock your leg, and I'm wondering if this rocking feels uncomfortable to you." Allow your client time and space to communicate. They might respond with, "no, it feels great! I didn't notice I was tensing up." From there you can work with that tensing response without having made an erroneous decision due to incorrect assumptions.

Best practices, universal precautions

So, in a world where anyone might be carrying trauma, should you walk on eggshells and avoid any behavior that might potentially trigger fear or guarding? No, you should be boldly yourself and offer your best work! And you should boldly accept your client for who they are, no matter how they communicate or respond to massage. Don't make assumptions based on how well you initially "click" or how well your first interactions go. Instead, present yourself for who you are, allow them to respond however they respond, and then do your best to meet their body and brain in the middle.

Here are some ways that I like to make my practice inviting to all, and to minimize the risk of harm in the case of past trauma:

1. **Lots of communication**. Take your time with the initial interview, and allow space and time for the client to tell their story. Whether or not you seem to get thorough and final answers, continue giving your client the opportunity to talk more during the massage and with each new session. Do more asking than telling, and remember the power differential (more on this in chapter 6).
2. **Create a safe space**. Thorough communication is the first step of this. Try not to leave questions in your client's mind about how undressed to get or when you'll be returning to the room. From there, be consistent with draping and be careful with drafts (keep the drape low as you work with it), and be aware of your finger direction as you work around potentially sensitive areas. Let everything you do communicate safety.
3. **Be willing to give up your agenda**. No matter what plan you formulate during the initial intake, be willing to throw it in the trash and start over from scratch if it doesn't seem to fit your client. In other words, don't come up with a template and try to force your client into it, but rather be adaptive to your

client. That might mean dropping trigger point work if a client finds it unpleasant, or moving to side-lying if a client finds being prone uncomfortable. For some clients, it might mean giving a massage unlike any that you've ever given before!

As an example, let's think about the anterior neck. You've got a client in your office with pronounced forward head posture who has been having jaw pain and temporal headaches. You've got good reason to believe that she'd be well-served by extensive work with the anterior and lateral neck muscles because this has been true for other clients, and because it follows a familiar pattern of referred pain.

During the intake, you ask about working with the anterior neck, pointing the area out on your own body. The client looks like she might have misgivings, so you elaborate: "This might feel weird, but it shouldn't be uncomfortable or painful. If it is, we'll back off and avoid the area. Would that be alright?" She agrees in a way that seems less tentative, so you proceed.

You work with the neck and shoulders broadly, warming the area and acclimating the client to your touch. Before you contact the anterior neck, you make sure to communicate that fact so that there are no surprises: "Okay Jane, I'd like to make contact with this ropey muscle that runs down the front and side of your neck. This can be a funky sensation, but it shouldn't be uncomfortable. Is that okay?"

A quick note: As you ask for informed consent and give people a heads up about working with sensitive areas, make sure not to accidentally poison the well by using prejudicial language. Stick to clinical and brief questions rather than using language that communicates that "this will be scary" or "this will suck." Don't belabor the point by saying that "some people really freak out when I work here" or "this might feel invasive." Yes, be honest and open, but don't prime people to feel fear about their own body.

Back to Jane: Despite your communication efforts and your attempts to acclimate the general area to touch, you notice that she seems to be in distress as you contact her sternocleidomastoid. It's subtle, but because you're tracking her face and her breathing, you notice that she has a slight grimace, and she seems to be holding her breath. You gently disengage from the SCM work and address the issue: "So it looked to me like you were having some discomfort during that, is that true for you?" Jane responds that it "felt a little like choking." She might be a little embarrassed about it, or even seem to be overall anxious about the entire incident. You say, "in that case, let's skip that front of the neck work, there's plenty of other useful work that we can do instead."

I'd like to acknowledge that this can be scary for you, the massage therapist. It's somewhat jarring to try a technique that you've used a hundred times to good effect and find that someone can't tolerate it, or even finds it anxiety-provoking. It's like eating a spoonful of sugar and discovering that it's actually salt. It can also be frustrating – you're sure that this client would benefit from this work, and now you're working with one hand tied behind your back!

I ask that you let all of that go. That feeling of jarring disconnect between what you intended and how a client received it? You communicated well, your client is unharmed, and you can let it go. That frustration of not being able to employ your best tools? Think of it as an opportunity to experiment with different approaches (there are plenty of ways to deal with forward head posture without ever touching the anterior neck!) and let it go.

Meet your client where they are, err on the side of too much communication, and let the outcome take care of itself.

On emotional releases

One day you might be working with a client and notice that they are making little noises that are hard to identify, or that they're tightening up all over. After a moment, you realize that the client is doing their best to keep from crying. This might stay subtle, or spill over into full on, body wracking sobs.

In the massage world, this is often called an "emotional release," with some teachers claiming that memory or trauma is stored in the body and able to be released by the right kind of contact. I find this unlikely. What's more likely is that the body is acting like a mnemonic device (a memory tool), and that interacting with certain parts in certain ways can evoke memory powerfully, often in ways that merely thinking or talking about the past is unable to do. It's like smelling baking bread and being struck by a vivid memory of your grandmother, even decades after her passing.

In the case of clients with past trauma, this can result in them reconnecting with a traumatic event suddenly and unintentionally. Some clients will feel grief or fear. For other clients, their tears might be from a strong and sudden feeling of relief, safety, or interpersonal connection. They may laugh instead of cry, or find themselves unable to stop shaking.

If you find yourself as the massage therapist in any of these situations, realize that there's nothing you need to do. It can feel unsettling and incongruous to go from gently vibing to sudden sobbing, but it's not something you did wrong, and it's not something you need to fix. Instead, I invite you to take an easy breath, take a mental step back, and let the client lead the way.

Start by either gradually removing your hands from the body and placing a supportive hand on the client's shoulder, or just slow your work down and stay where you are. From there, ask, "Hey Jane, how are you doing? Would you like me to stop for a bit, or should I keep working?" The client might prefer a break, or that you keep at it. As you do so, offer your support: "Let me know if you need anything. Can I grab you a tissue, or some water?"

Merely by being calm and supportive, you're accomplishing everything that your client is likely to need in that moment. A sudden emotional outpouring can be jarring for the client, and even a little embarrassing. It can feel like an unwanted loss of control. In that moment, the most welcome thing in the world is a massage therapist who doesn't seem the least bit freaked out, and who seems to have seen it all before.

As the wave of emotion passes, you'll probably be able to start working again (ask beforehand, and make sure it's fine to work on the area that coincided with the release), and from there it's just a matter of everyone breathing and getting back into the massage. The client might apologize, so reassure them that this is something that happens sometimes, and it's okay if it happens again.

Relax, don't do it

The upshot of this interlude: You're likely to encounter people living with trauma, and it doesn't mean you need to be a trauma expert. Communicate, be willing to give up an agenda or technique that isn't working, and make your environment and your touch safe and supportive.

There is an exception, though. I have a "don't" that I'd like to include with my "dos." Don't order people to relax. Don't order people to breathe. Even if this way of interacting with clients has worked a thousand times before, and even if this is how your teachers talked to you, don't order your clients to do anything.

If a client's arm is seized up with tension, saying the word "relax" as a complete sentence might seem natural, and like a reasonable thing for a massage therapist to say. I'd just like you to keep in mind how these words of soothing are often weaponized by abusers. A parent screaming "relax!" at their child while physically restraining them during a crying jag. A man telling his partner to "just breathe!" while being the one who provoked the panic.

Ordering someone to relax has never once been relaxing in the history of language, and yet the tradition persists.

What can you do if you can't say, "relax"? You can say more words along with it, and you can choose to make it a request rather than a command. For me, that sounds like this: "See if you can relax your shoulder muscles as I move your arm," or "I'm going to be moving your head around just a little bit. Try to be as loosey goosey as possible and allow those neck muscles to stay relaxed."

This can apply to asking your clients to do active engagement, to having them speak up about pain, and pretty much every situation where their help is optional. These phrases can be useful: "If you'd like to," "if it feels right for you," "feel free to."

And now, consider broadening that philosophy to everything about your massage. Your every contact can be a silent question: "Is this alright? Do I still have your permission?" By placing your hands confidently but slowly, you can continue the process of asking for consent as you work.

Let every session be new

Finally, as part and parcel of stepping away from adherence to an agenda, be willing to let go of old preconceptions about what your client is and isn't able to handle. If you have a client in your office who came for work with their PTSD symptoms, or a client who has preferences or behaviors that once prevented you from working in certain ways, realize that these conditions can change over time. Hold on to what you've learned during your therapeutic relationship, but be willing to let go of old approaches if they no longer seem necessary. One day, your client might be able to give up control of that arm, or place their head in that face cradle. Communication can help ease these transitions, or they might happen organically and wordlessly.

Before I leave this section, I want to give a shout out to the massage therapists out there who are living with post-traumatic stress. Your work might sometimes interact with your experience of trauma in unpleasant or unusual ways, and all I ask is that you extend yourself the same grace and non-judgment that you offer your clients. Don't think that you always need to be in just the right headspace to be a good therapist, or that you always need to push through when you're feeling overwhelmed. Take care of yourself, make the changes you need to be comfortable, and let every session be new.

Chapter 5: I'm the One in Pain!

Having pain as a massage therapist sucks. Not only does it affect your happiness and mental health as you do your job, it can make you question your worth as a bodywork professional. Surely I should be able to cure myself! Surely I should be able to massage this away, or figure out better ways to apply techniques. Am I not using proper body mechanics? Do I need to be even more strict with my straight back and stacked joints?!

I've got good news: The answer *probably* isn't to become more scrupulous about moving perfectly or standing perfectly. For most massage therapists in pain, you don't need to beat yourself up about sloppy posture, and you don't need to give up doing the techniques you love in order to be pain free.

The body isn't a ticking time bomb waiting to blow the moment you make a mistake and slouch too much. No, the body is resilient and adaptable, able to reinforce itself in ways that let people participate in World's Strongest Man competitions, or do 1080s on a skateboard, or stay bent for ten-hour days picking crops. Yes, each of these endeavors can come with their own share of pain, but that's an important lesson:

Injuries happen. Pain accumulates, or sometimes seems to spike out of nowhere. We tell ourselves that we can avoid pain if only we "act right," but that's a fallacy. The world is much messier than that, and trying to block all possible avenues of injury or insult only leaves us severely constricted, trapped in a padded bubble that, eventually, kind of hurts.

What I'm trying to say is that you should expect occasional pain and dysfunction, whether it's from doing 25 hours of hands-on work every week, or your daily yoga practice, or just from sleeping (and no, you don't need to "sleep wrong" to occasionally wake up with a new ache). One time I was standing perfectly still in the shower and my back decided to spasm. And I promise I wasn't showering wrong, or using poor shower body mechanics!

Pain patterns

That isn't to say that pain is completely random and that we should just give in to constant and recurring injury. No, pain tends to follow distinct patterns based on activity, and there are ways to reduce the likelihood of injury, as well as each episode's intensity and duration. You've probably noticed this in your clients: Office workers have different patterns of pain than hair stylists, who have different patterns than veterinarians or construction workers.

Let's talk about office workers. When I think of my desk-bound clients, I see a lot of protraction and flexion – in other words, these people spend their days curled forward and inward, and their pain patterns follow from this. They're more likely to have wrist and arm issues, including numbness at night, that can be associated with nerve impingement near the shoulder. They're more likely to have tight hip flexors and external rotators, with attendant low back pain and glute numbness. Headaches at the base of the skull aren't unusual, nor are tight and sensitive upper traps. When I think of treating someone with any or all of the above symptoms, I want to encourage retraction and extension, and reduce the tug-of-war tension that's keeping those traps so tight.

What about massage therapists? Here's what I've seen in my MT clients, and in myself:

- Arm pain and shoulder dysfunction, often with numbness at night. Upper back pain and tightness. We spend long hours with our arms in front of our bodies, pressing forward and down. This results in strong pecs pulling us into protraction, with the traps and rhomboids desperately trying to stay strong in this extended position.
- Wrist pain, often centered on the pisiform bone (the pokey little carpal on the ulnar side of your wrist). Sometimes there will be pain that feels deep within the joint. I associate this with frequent use of the carpal region to apply pressure, usually with the wrist brought slightly into hyperextension.

- Thumb pain, often at the metacarpophalangeal joint. I associate this with lots of squeezing and stripping using the thumbs.
- All manner of hip and low back pain. Massage therapists sometimes pick a favorite posture and stick with it for five or eight hours a day, even if it becomes tiresome and achy halfway through.

There might also be headaches and foot pain and neck pain. Some massage therapists lose track of their heads and spend hours every day with it cocked to one side, or hanging forward as they try to use x-ray vision on their clients. So, surely it's time to straighten up and fly right, right?

The prescription for perfection

Shoulders back, head upright! Strong low back, butt stuck out! No wrist extension, never use your thumbs! Heck, let's stop using those hands altogether and only use forearms!

Wait... that causes pain too? Now you've got tension headaches and low back pain and ulnar nerve irritation? Crap. Well, try standing straighter, and never look at your client, and... Yes, as you can tell, this can be a never-ending task. If you ask about your massage-related pain on message boards, or talk to continuing education teachers or colleagues, you might hear a lot about how the pain is your fault, and how you could be pain-free if only you were perfect.

Or at least, that's the message that underlies most talk of body mechanics in the massage world: There is a right way, and you're not doing it. Those other people who say they have the right way are wrong. You'll have people chiming in and saying that you should abandon the massage that you learned in school entirely and use this tool, or switch to Thai massage, or switch to using your feet.

"But Ian, aren't you saying that they're wrong and you're right, and you know the one true path to correct body mechanics?" No, I'm saying they're *all correct* about good ways to use the body for massage, *all at the same time*! They're just wrong about the prescription.

One size fits none

I am, and this is putting it kindly, lanky. My arms are so long that I have difficulty finding dress shirts that fit (ever notice how I always have my sleeves rolled up in my videos, even when I'm not working on a client?). I've got mild pectus excavatum so I *stay* curled forward. My feet are so flat they could be defined by three points on graph paper, and they point out to either side like I've got two places to be.

The standard advice for body mechanics has never felt right to me, especially after a long day of massage. I quickly find any sort of strict posture painful, and the power stances and hip shifting would leave me sweating within minutes. It all just felt so effortful and forced to me.

Part of this is the natural adaptation process to new ways of moving. If you're a student or new massage therapist and you find yourself wiped out by a day of work, realize that there is a lot of transformation left in you, and you will discover that previously difficult workloads eventually become easy. Your hands will strengthen, certain aches will subside, and your body will reinforce you as you move forward.

But, if you're like me, you might come to the conclusion that these prescriptions are too strict, and some of them are made for someone else's body. You might have already noticed that you sometimes need to change techniques to account for the length of your arms or the size of your chest. You might have felt like it was impossible to generate power in certain positions, so you either "broke the rules" or you powered through with the strength of your arms and hands. This can eventually lead to strain and fatigue — wouldn't it be nice to feel comfort and ease instead?

Finding your body mechanics

If the body mechanics you're using are serving you well, then skip this chapter and do so with my blessing. If it ain't broke, don't fix it.

If you're still in massage school, I encourage you to use your teachers' body mechanics recommendations when and if you're able. These will be new ways of moving, and even if some of them feel awkward or tiring at first, that could just be part of the growth process. Talk to them about it if you ever feel unsure whether what you're feeling is normal. And if it ever comes down to listening to me or listening to your teacher, I'd prefer that while you're in massage school, you really immerse yourself in massage school. There's a lot of valuable technique and knowledge to discover, even if you end up eventually discarding parts of it. That goes for continuing education classes as well; even if some of it ends up being dubious, there's always treasure to be found. Dive in, have the full experience, and worry about separating the wheat from the chaff later.

But once you've applied massage for a few hundred hours and you've got a sense of what works for you and what feels like a poor fit, it's time to do some experimentation. Realize that you won't always have an "ah ha!" moment when you hit upon a useful new way of moving; just like in massage school, it will likely feel awkward at first and require some time before you can really determine whether it's right for your body.

So, my prescription for body mechanics: Be playful, but persistent. Try out lots of ways to move, and either stick with them long enough to see whether they have value for you, or be willing to try them again after a while. Here are some things to try:

Play with table height. This is easiest with an electric table that you can raise and lower at will (an excellent investment!), but you can also try this in short bursts with a willing partner, or try small incremental changes throughout your workday. My main advice here is to try a lower table than you're used to. This might initially feel more tiring than a higher table, with fatigue in your back and hips.

This can be prevented by taking advantage of the new angle and throwing your weight around. Now that you're higher up relative to your client, you can shift your upper body *over* their body and lean in with straight limbs. Techniques that used to take muscular effort from your triceps and shoulders can now be applied just by placing your hands, leaning, and letting gravity do the work.

Interact with the table. In massage school you might have been told to stand away from the table to avoid any possible interaction with the client's body. If so, consider throwing that advice into a bonfire.

The massage table, especially once it's been lowered a bit, can be a valuable source of support and leverage as you work. Rather than using your back as a crane and always expecting it to bear the weight of your return to an upright posture, you can lean a thigh against the side of the table, using it to stabilize your body as you step, lunge, lean, and reset.

Try placing a hand or fist on the surface of the massage table as you work using the other arm. This can allow you to sink your weight down into the table while only giving some of it to the client. You can also shift your weight far above your client by planting a knee on the table and giving yourself some extra height.

You can use your feet to bolster body parts, you can sit next to a side-lying client to stabilize their hips, or place a knee next to a leg that wants to externally rotate. As you experiment with using more of your body to interact with the table and with your client, remember to communicate: "John, I'd like to stabilize your knee using the side of my body. Would that be alright? Okay great, just let me know if I'm ever too far into your personal space." In other words, keep consent and comfort in mind as you experiment.

Break the posture rules. I know you're supposed to keep your shoulders down and back, and your lumbar spine curved, and you're supposed to sink into a lunge or squat while generating power with your legs, but what if you... didn't? At least sometimes?

What if you tucked your tailbone as you leaned your hip into the table, and slouched your shoulders as you poured your upper body weight into your client? Not the whole time, but sometimes.

What if you had a seat on your stool while working with your client's rotator cuff or lateral hip? What advantages would that new angle have, and how could you generate power in that position?

Dance and have fun! Imagine a massage session where you really allowed yourself to get into the music. There would be long sweeping effleurage, and quick vigorous petrissage. As you compressed a point on the scapula, you wouldn't be able to stop yourself from moving your head and your hips. As you rock out, you could also rock your client's low back and limbs. Would that be a worse massage than if you had kept "perfect" posture and used no extraneous motion?

Of course not! The best massages are the ones where there's flow and experimentation and a sense of play. If you've felt stagnant and locked into your routine for so long that it's kind of driving you crazy, then it's time to start moving in new and different ways. Even if you have to listen to your standard spa music, you can still choose to groove on it.

If you'd like a prescription for the "best" body mechanics, here's what I've got: **Stay in touch with your body, and make changes before fatigue sets in**. You can use your thumbs, you can use your wrists, and you can angle your head. Just be mindful as you do so, and have enough variety built into your sessions that no single part of you ever starts feeling tired. If you've got a shoulder routine that you and your clients love, but your thumbs feel kind of tired or even achy by the end of it, then you might be setting yourself up for trouble. Either break that routine into smaller parts, or find more excuses to use other tools like knuckles, forearms, and fists.

Injury prevention for massage athletes

The first step to having less pain as a massage therapist is to realize that you are an *athlete*. You do a very specialized physical activity for many hours a week, often involving the repetition of specific and rather idiosyncratic movements that aren't found in any other field of medicine or sport. If you compress the pec major laterally while moving the arm into external rotation 4-6 times on every client, you've done it hundreds of times by the end of the week! That's not even considering all the cranial cradles and trapezius squeezes and hip compressions. By the time you're working with 80 clients per month, you're giving your body ample reason to make adaptations specific to your unique line of work.

And adaptation is good! Your body will strengthen your pecs to help you press forward and down; your forearm flexors and extensors will bulk up for maximal stability; your trunk, hips, and legs will tighten up and strengthen to keep you standing and lunging for 6 hours out of the day; and your feet and ankles will tighten and get reinforced with extra collagen until... ouch! How the heck did I end up with plantar fasciitis?!

Or it could be any of the above: Your newly strengthened forearms might be yanking on your newly reinforced tendons in a way that irritates your median nerve, and suddenly you've got the symptoms of carpal tunnel syndrome. Your shoulder girdle muscles, which are now more than capable of bracing your arms for hours of forward compression, might start to clamp down on the brachial plexus at all hours of the day, causing numbness as you try to sleep at night. That trunk and hip tightness, which are so useful to keep you effortlessly standing for hours per day, could end up feeling like low back pain, or even sciatica.

We'll talk more about specific ways to deal with common massage therapists' injuries in a moment, but before we do that, I want you to zoom way out. This isn't about one body part malfunctioning in a way that no one could have predicted; injury is entirely predictable when you're asking a lot of the body, and then doing one activity over and over again! That's called an overuse injury, or a repetitive stress injury (RSI), and every specialized field has its own constellation of RSIs. What can you do to avoid this? I want you to do what any high-level athlete would do to reduce the frequency of injury and to get better at their sport at the same time: *Cross-train.*

I know that a full week of massage can leave you feeling pretty wiped out, but letting massage be your only form of physical activity is a trap, and it's one that can shorten your career. By repeatedly and persistently giving only one kind of stimulus to your body, you're sending a powerful signal that you need some specific alterations to how your body works. You need your hamstrings to stay a certain length and no longer; you need your calves to be tight and for your ankles to never do much flexion in either direction; you need tight rotator cuffs, and your arms pretty much never need to go above your head. Your body, the ever-attentive listener, will make these changes faithfully. And by the end of the process, you'll be in a box of your own creation, surrounded by tight, irritable muscle that's ready to start reporting pain at any moment.

It might seem crazy when you're tired and achy, but the answer to this contraction of possibilities is *more* activity, not less. If your body is tight and prone to headache and upper back spasms, imagine what the body must think when you implement a morning yoga routine three days per week. Suddenly it's being asked to do very different movements than it's used to, with the ankles in pronounced dorsiflexion and plantar flexion, and the arms high above the head, and the thigh extended far back behind the pelvis. As these new stimuli are sent regularly and repeatedly, the spinal cord adapts to the new reality, allowing the hamstrings to go further into extension, and the arms to reach to the sky as rotator cuff tension is reduced. It will now try to strengthen your body for a much wider range of activities, expanding and empowering all at once.

And it doesn't have to be yoga! All sorts of cardio can convince your body to stay loose and flexible while damping down sensitivity. Running, swimming, rowing, biking: All great. But as you consider what to add to your cross-training regimen, look for opportunities to introduce stimuli that are completely unlike your hours of massage. Tack on a stretching routine after your runs, lengthening those hip flexors and broadening those pecs. Do some jumping jacks and cartwheels after you're gone biking. Dance around in your living room, eventually perfecting the routine from Napoleon Dynamite down to the very last detail.

Finally, consider weight training. As far as injury prevention goes, this is my number one recommendation: Convince your body to pack on a little extra muscle mass. If you get tired doing squats and lunges during your fifth session of the day, consider how much easier things would feel if you're used to having 100+ pounds on your upper back as you squat. If your lower back gets tight as your day wears on, think about how much stronger it would feel if you frequently do deadlifts and weighted crunches. The same goes for your forearms, shoulders, and calves. Rather than waiting around to see how those areas adapt to long hours of massage, show them how you'd like them to adapt by giving them big stimuli!

This is also a way of introducing new movements that you won't encounter in your massage office, and even exercises meant to counteract your most frequent movements. In other words, since you do a lot of pressing forward, make sure your weight training routine involves plenty of pulling back and pressing overhead. Because you're bent forward for much of the day, do moves that ask you to stand tall and extend your hips.

Not sure where to start? This is a job for a personal trainer or athletic trainer. You can use the programs offered at most gyms, or seek out independent trainers who have lots of experience and convincing credentials. Any trainer worth their salt will be able to get you started with a routine tailored to your fitness level and the needs of your body, as well as help you respond to any difficulty or discomfort you might encounter.

Just say no to pressure junkies

Another way of preventing injuries is to know your current limits, and to communicate these clearly to your clients. Repeatedly, if need be. You see, in the course of your career you'll come across the type of person who says this: "Just dig in as hard as you can! I'm not happy unless you're making me cry." Oh dear, it's the *pressure junky*.

I've never known quite how people reach this state, but here's how I imagine their origin story played out: They went in for their first massage, and their massage therapist really laid into them. Elbows deep into trigger points, stripping muscles while asking for eccentric contraction, telling them to "just breathe" while they're already huffing and puffing from pain. Some clients will be completely turned off (and even injured) by this rough treatment, while others will leave the room with their body coursing with endorphins and a new philosophy of self-care: If it hurts, it works.

This is usually the same type of person who glories in having "the worst knots" or "the tightest shoulders" their past massage therapists had ever felt (side note: Please don't say things like this to clients). In other words, pain is a competition, injury is a gold medal, and they're playing to win.

Just realize that you don't need to participate in any part of this process. You don't need to compete with their past therapists, you don't need to take it as a challenge when they say things like, "you can't hurt me," and you don't need to buy into the philosophy of pain as care. Indeed, it's your job as the expert on massage in the room to try to bring this client on board with a body-friendly approach. That can sound something like this: "Joe, it sounds like you're used to painful massage, but I find that I get the best results when I stop short of the point of physical discomfort. I'd like to work with your body in a way that feels good, because I think that's an indication that I'm working *with* your nervous system rather than against it. Is that something you'd be willing to try?"

This can work, and I'd say that about half the time I can get these clients to try my quasi-myofascial approach and leave them just as satisfied as they were with the painful work. But sometimes they'll immediately object with something like, "I'm here for deep tissue, so go ahead and dig in!" or they'll just keep asking for more pressure once they're on the table. In these cases, if a client is asking to be hurt and encouraging you to do dangerous things with your joints, it's time to put your foot down, both as a matter of professional ethics, and to preserve your own body. That can sound like this: "This is actually my maximum pressure. Will that work for you?"

And if it's not enough, then stop the session, give them the name of a massage therapist who loves digging in, and go on with your day. I recommend not charging, as this is likely just as frustrating for them as it was for you. Going forward, this problem can be prevented by talking more about your massage philosophy on your website and social media outlets, or by having your front desk workers direct pressure junkies to a better fit.

Here's what I don't want you to do: Don't try to be everything to everyone. Don't try to compete with that other massage therapist for the title of World's Strongest. Just because a client is asking for something, that doesn't make it the right call, especially if your health and happiness are at risk.

I once had a client who asked me to work very deeply, specifically asking that I use my thumbs to do so. I complied, because I had a head full of porridge and the deep-seated need to please everyone. I felt a twinge during that massage that turned into an injury, and it took the better part of a year to rehabilitate. Learn from young, porridge-headed Ian!

What to do when you've got pain

If you find yourself with developing pain, there are some changes you can make and some self-care that you can implement to help shepherd those twinges and injuries back to a happier existence:

1. The first step in rehabilitating any injury is to stop aggravating it. This can be hard when pain seems to come out of nowhere, but look at your work habits and your usual massage routine and try to identify possible suspects. From there, experiment with different ways of moving and find modifications that seem less likely to exacerbate your pain. These changes can be temporary, but make a note of what works for you in case that particular pain rears its head again in the future.
2. Soothe yourself. After work, apply your favorite pain reduction and nervous system soothing techniques to your injured part. For pain centered on a joint, I prefer ice and an Ace bandage wrap. For muscle spasm and tightness, I like heat. You might be trained in kinesiotaping, or know a skilled acupuncturist. Whatever you choose, apply it on a regular basis, and let that part rest.

3. Gradually introduce exercise and massage. Once your pain is no longer acute and you're not at risk of spasm, start using that part of your body in new ways. Strengthen and stretch, and use your favorite massage techniques (or go get a massage!) to work with the area and everything connected to it.
4. Start using the part again. Once your pain has mostly passed, you can experiment with undoing some of the initial changes that you made to prevent aggravation. A previously injured part doesn't need to be protected forever — indeed, getting it back to work can be an essential part of the healing process. Feel free to avoid a prior approach that wasn't working for you, but trust your own resilience and adaptability.

One big caveat here: If your pain is persistent, severe, or interfering with your ability to work or live your life, then go see your doctor. They can evaluate your injury and refer you to a specialist if need be. If your pain is purely musculoskeletal, ask to be referred to a physical therapist or occupational therapist. They'll be able to design a stretching, strengthening, and soothing regimen just for you.

How to deal with various aches and injuries

Let's get specific. As we talk about the various injuries that are common among massage therapists, remember that nothing here is one-size-fits-all, and that you may need to make changes for your own unique body. Again, if your pain is severe or if you're having trouble implementing a self-care regimen, go see your doctor or physical therapist. All the tools and exercises mentioned below can be seen by going to massagesloth.com/booksupplement.

Thumb pain. This is common among massage therapists, and it's usually felt at the base of the thumb (either the metacarpophalangeal joint or the carpometacarpal joint). It tends to result from using the thumbs for lots of petrissage over the course of every massage, as well as using the thumbs to strip tissue or compress trigger points. These are all fine techniques, but their frequency and duration should be limited until your thumbs are happy. Give yourself a thumb vacation by reducing or eliminating thumb use completely for a couple of weeks, finding other ways to squeeze and lift tissues. Experiment with lots of fist and forearm work.

Start a daily regimen of ice plunges after work: Immerse your entire hand and forearm in a container of ice water; hold until numb or you can't stand it, then remove and towel dry. Repeat, then wrap with an Ace bandage. Keep using your thumb for daily tasks around the house, but avoid anything that directly aggravates your pain.

As pain subsides, institute a regimen of strengthening using therapy putty and extension exercises (I like Expand-your-hands rubber bands from IronMind for this purpose, which you can find on Amazon). Start with low resistance and listen to your body — some pain during the exercise is okay, but if your pain flares up substantially during or after the session, then use less resistance or lower duration. Follow with light stretching and an ice water plunge.

After a week or two of exercise, gradually reintroduce your thumbs to your massage work. As you do so, be mindful of what positions feel powerful and supported, and which feel vulnerable. Use positions of strength when possible, and support your thumbs in weaker positions (e.g., using two thumbs instead of one; adding fingers nearby when using for fine work; sometimes taking the thumb out of petrissage and instead using the fingers to compress tissue against your palm). Remember all of the new moves that you implemented during your thumb vacation, and use those for a greater proportion of the massage, even as your thumbs fully recover.

Wrist pain. This might be felt deep in the joint at all times or only upon extension, or at the little pisiform bone on the ulnar side of the wrist. This is most common when the carpal region is used as a primary massage tool, especially when the wrist is in extension bordering on hyperextension. In other words, you've found that you can apply lots of body weight using just your carpal bones, and you're spending a lot of each session doing so.

Start with a wrist vacation. This is more difficult than a thumb vacation because it's difficult to take the wrist completely out of the picture, but experiment with ways to spend less of each session with your carpals doing the work. Add forearms for more of the session, use fingertips, use fists. If you want to use the palmar surface of your hand, do so with the other hand stacked on top. Keep an eye out for motions that cause wrist pain, and try to work around them until your sensitivity and pain subside.

Daily ice water plunges are a good idea here, followed by either an Ace bandage or a wrist brace (I remove the rigid plate so that I can have the compression without the immobilization). Keep using your hands for your daily tasks, but keep an eye out for anything that causes your pain to flare.

As your pain subsides, start a daily regimen of stretching, strengthening, and massage. Use the therapy putty and finger extension bands as above, along with wrist flexion and extension exercises. These can be done with free weights, a wrist roller (a bar with a cord that you use to reel in a weight using flexion and extension), or a Thera-band Flexbar. Once you have fatigued your hands and forearms, do some gentle stretching of the wrist flexors and extensors, with your wrist both prone and supine. Do an ice plunge, dry off, and wrap or splint.

You can do massage as part of the above regimen (as a warm-up prior to the exercise, for example) or separately. For this, I like using an open fist to slowly iron out the flexors and extensors. You might be tempted to dig in on points that seem extra sensitive or on the wrist itself — and feel free to experiment! — but my watchword is "soothing." Let's get this high-tension, high-sensitivity wrist situation to chill out.

As you reimplement more palmar contact, be aware of how you're applying that palm. If you're unconsciously sinking in with the heel of hand, that can be stressful for that joint, and it can be sharper than you intend. If you mean to use a nice broad palm, then allow the entire surface to apply pressure rather than just the carpals. The heel of hand is a nice tool, just use it conscientiously!

Neck pain and stiffness; headaches. I group these together because they probably come from the same source: Bunched up shoulders held tight, and the neck jutted forward. This can feel like a position of power because it does bolster the shoulder joints while giving you a slightly higher vantage for downward pressure. Having your neck forward can feel like you're allowing yourself to relax, but it's often a symptom of trying to use x-ray vision on a body part, or finding a retracted neck posture tiresome after 5 hours.

If you'd like to give your neck and shoulders a break, this is a job for mindfulness. Keep a mental eye out for when your shoulders start to creep up and monitor the tone in your upper trapezius. Watch your head position and see if you can catch yourself allowing it to jut forward, or keeping it cocked to the side for prolonged periods. Once you've got a better idea of when you're engaging in these behaviors and for how long, you can choose to introduce variety.

Allow your shoulders to drop and retract. Allow your neck to be long and erect, retracting your chin. Feel how these positions change your internal sensation of tension in your own body and watch for when they become fatiguing. And then, introduce more variety! You can bunch those shoulders and cock that head. You can make that neck retraction more or less strict. As you play with these positions over the course of your day, find what works for you, and allow a new normal where there's less unconscious bunching and jutting and more variety in how you hold your body. Being mindful of these things can be a lot of work at first, but it gets easier and more automatic over time.

As for treatments for this pain: If you've got a crick in the neck (painful and limited rotation to one or both sides), don't try to stretch your way out of this situation. Instead, be patient, try heat or ice — or alternate between the two — and wait for the acute period to subside. You can do gentle stretches of the levator scapulae after this, but my favorite low-impact, low-stress exercise for cricks, neck pain, and headache are gentle neck retractions. A few repetitions of chin tucks between clients can remind your neck that it can easily rest with more posterior length rather than staying all bunched up.

For all shoulder/neck/head/upper back pain, consider the pecs. When I think of a massage therapist with upper torso pain and bunched up traps, I'm imagining powerful pecs and stressed-out rhomboids along with them. So! Institute some stretches that elongate the pecs and engage the rhomboids, drawing the shoulders back and down. Institute some resistance training that engages the shoulder retractors and depressors, with bent-over rows, back flyes, and pull-ups all being excellent add-ons to your existing routine.

Finally, consider the position of your table. If you're bunching your shoulders to bolster yourself for powerful work at the height of your abdomen or sternum, consider dropping your client lower! If your client is at waist-height or lower, you can more easily drop those shoulders, lean forward, and let gravity drive your work. Your shoulders will thank you, and your techniques will feel more like a force of nature.

Low back and hip pain. If you find yourself with more than your share of low back and hip problems that seem to flare up after a long day at work, my main suspect is what I call "using your back as a crane." That's where your torso is far out in front of your hips (maybe at the end of an effleurage stroke up the leg), and you haul yourself back to standing using your hip and trunk extensors. There might also be some side-bending involved, with quadratus lumborum being expected to be long and strong as you bring yourself from slumped to standing over and over again.

My second suspect is that you're in the habit of losing your legs. It's been a long five hours of work so far and you've got two more to go. You started the day doing lunges and squats, but as your legs fatigued, you accidentally started standing taller and letting yourself bend from the butt and spine rather than using bent knees as your base.

Standing tall is fine, as is slumping against the table, as are squats and lunges. What I ask is that you use your body mindfully, and that you keep an eye on what you do to purposely add variety, and what you're mindlessly falling into as a response to fatigue. It's in that sixth hour of hands-on work when this will have the most impact: Have you been listening to your body this whole time and making changes before fatigue sets in? Or have you already pushed past fatigue about ten times and now there's nothing left in the tank for your big finish? It's in this latter scenario where injury can easily take place.

So, let's make some changes. Only use your back as a crane in specific circumstances, and recognize it as a power move rather than just another way of ending an effleurage stroke. I do this when I've got my hands on either side of my client's QL region and I'm scooping up toward the sky, dragging that lumbar fascia with me. I start with my butt stuck out, I'm plastered against the side of the table in a lunge position, and I stand up with tight abs, dragging the client's lateral tissue with me. I recognize that I'm engaging my spinal erectors and hip extensors, and I keep an eye out for any fatigue. Because I do these power moves so infrequently (have I mentioned that I'm lazy?), this just feels like a nice change of pace and a chance to work muscles that have mostly been relaxed for the past hour.

What about when you need to stand up from a reaching move? First, reach less. If you're doing a long move up the leg while starting at the ankle, follow that stroke with your body. You can do this by shuffling your feet, or by taking a tai chi step. That means keeping your foot low and allowing it to flow just over the ground, placing it gently and firmly as you shift your weight. Or you can just take a big plodding step. Do what feels right, and do what preserves your stamina. Second, use your client's body or the table to help you stand. Whether you follow your stroke with your body or not, you can choose to press yourself back up to standing by walking your hands back toward yourself. These can be compressive techniques or effleurage, or you can just sink a palm into the table as you come back to your center. Play around with different ways of getting back to an upright position after a long technique, and use a variety of approaches.

If you've got acute low back pain (i.e., you felt a twinge and now things are locked up), that's a job for rest. In other words, I recommend against trying to stretch or massage an area in spasm. Instead, take baby steps to your favorite chair, lean back on a heating pad, and let time do its work. You can switch out heat for ice every half hour or so if you'd like to see how your body responds to contrast therapy. As your pain becomes stiffness over the next day or so, continue your heat/ice therapy and gradually introduce cat cow stretches, starting with a small range of motion.

For chronic low back pain, meaning frequent stiffness or aches that flare up after a long day or when you're trying to get to sleep at night, institute a regimen of stretching and strengthening. Something as simple as a 15-minute morning yoga routine could be all you need, and you could also let your body know that it's time to bolster your hips and your core with extra muscle. To strengthen your hips, that's a job for squats, lunges, and deadlifts, preferably under the initial supervision of a qualified trainer. The machines at your gym can do a good job, as can bodyweight squats and lunges.

Doing core work can help, meaning crunches and planks and the like. Just realize that these can also activate your hip flexors, which can be involved in low back and hip pain if allowed to stay short and sensitive. If you find your low back pain flaring after using an ab wheel, the hip flexors are a likely culprit. As you work with your hips and core, take some time to include lunge stretches, back bridges, upward facing dog poses, or other movements that remind your hip flexors that they are able to elongate.

When you get a massage, hip work will likely be your best bet for preventing future low back pain. Ask your massage therapist to iron out your hip extensors, external rotators, and abductors. You can also have them check in with iliacus and psoas (just tell them to be gentle!). If they seem determined to just attack the QL region, ask them to broaden their approach. You can also accomplish much of this yourself using a foam roller: Roll along your sacroiliac joint and all along your posterior and lateral ilium. Include your hamstrings and low back. Lie back with your feet on the ground and your knees pointed toward the ceiling, with the foam roller under your sacrum, and gently rock your knees from side to side.

Finally, play more when you're working. Find excuses to bend into a hamstring stretch as you sink into tissue, and go into extra deep lunges that stretch your hip flexors. Dance, do techniques "wrong," give the client some jostling and tapotement, etc. A monotonous, repetitive workday is the enemy of low backs everywhere, so treat yourself to a bit of mindful weirdness.

Foot pain. So, you've mostly dealt with the other aches and pains that can come from massage. You're varying your stance, you're using plenty of different hand and forearm configurations, and you're letting the table and the client take your weight rather than pressing or pulling (except sometimes, when you feel like it). But when all's said and done, you're still on your feet for six or more hours per day, and you're feeling it! This might be fatigue, or it might be pain in the foot, the heel, or the ankle. You might even have pain upon standing up from bed in the morning, like a shard of glass in the heel. That last symptom is a hallmark of plantar fasciitis, by the way. If it becomes severe or persistent, please see a physical therapist.

What to do with foot pain? It's not like we can just stop *standing* during our workday. Except... wait for it, some of you will know what I'm about to say: Why not sit more? Especially on longer days, why not find five minutes here and there to rest your feet, all while adding even more variety to your routine and to how you use your body?

Here's what this can look like: You're working on one side of a prone client's back, and you swoop up to their shoulder. After some nice petrissage of the trapezius and deltoid, you grab their forearm and draw it out past the edge of the table, guiding the arm into a comfortable abducted position with the forearm hanging down toward the floor. This opens the axilla and relaxes the superior traps, and it offers all sorts of possibilities for shoulder work from new angles. My favorite method is to have a seat and work from there!

Seated massage has some interesting advantages other than just resting your feet. You're able to apply pressure toward the lateral aspect of your client's body with much more leverage than if you tried to do so from standing. You're up close and personal with the lateral ribs, allowing you to use forearms to lift and mobilize the latissimus. You can roll your stool down toward their hips and press superiorly with your hands or forearms, pressing all that lateral rib tissue up toward the axilla. From there you can use both hands to petrissage the entire scapula, allowing your thumb pads to gently compress the subscapularis as you make a "scapula sandwich." There's plenty of great opportunity to work with the triceps, deltoid, and trapezius from this seated position as well. Sometimes I'll sit for a whole five minutes per side, really exploring that shoulder!

This new angle works well for other areas too, allowing you to give extra attention to the lateral aspects of the pelvis and thighs. You'll never have an easier time working with gluteus medius than when you're seated. Between these additions and the time spent seated while working with the neck and shoulders while the client is supine, you might find yourself rolling around on your stool for up to a third of the massage. That's a lot less demanding for your feet and calves, and it can also be a relief for your low back. In the end, adding bits and pieces of seated work is just another way to play with how you use your body during massage, so give it a try and see what feels right for you.

But what if your feet are already hurting? This is another application where I like ice baths, though a hot epsom salt foot bath would be great too. Whichever you choose, I recommend also having a daily calf stretching regimen (any lunge will stretch the calves, though you might have to shift a bit until you can feel it in the posterior leg), and giving your feet some daily massage. This can be as simple as throwing a golf ball under your favorite chair and rolling it around under your foot, which is easiest on carpet. Imagine the ball acting as a thumb and explore the ball of your foot, the lateral and medial arch, the heel, and everything in between. Do a quick two-minute session per foot as often as you like, give yourself foot baths when you feel like it, do some stretching and strengthening, and your feet should feel better in no time.

That's my secret, Captain. I'm always injured.

I've got something to admit: While I live a mostly pain-free life, I'm also constantly tweaking one muscle or another, or winding up with joint pain in new and exciting places. This is despite my best efforts at having perfect posture while doing massage or running or doing deadlifts. Even with all my research into technique and my knowledge of biomechanics, I still wind up with aches and pains, some of them more persistent than others. My massage career has taught me how to limit these problems and reduce their intensity and duration, but not how to eliminate them completely.

While there might be some absolutely bullet-proof person whose next level body mechanics have made them invincible, I haven't met them. I've worked on many massage therapists, and I haven't encountered one who was immune to the occasional injury.

And my friends, that's life. Ignore the gurus who sell a vision of life without pain or suffering. Life is messy, progress is never linear, and recovery usually involves relapse.

The body, in all its elegance and resilience, is also a chaotic dance of trillions of cells forming a complex arrangement of pulleys and weights, monitored by nervous system inputs that actively compete to determine who gets heard and what gets done. We think of homeostasis as the body in balance, but it's actually the balance of multiple systems in balance, all of which are made up of many small balancing acts. And it can all go awry if a single neuron breaks through the threshold of excitation and says, "hey, there's danger in this specific multifidus muscle! Better lock things down until we figure out what's going on!"

We try to make life so clean and comprehensible. If someone goes to jail, they must have been a villain. If someone gets sick, they must have lived recklessly. If someone gets hurt, there must have been a way to prevent it.

But we all know better. Sometimes innocent people get punished, and sometimes people get sick for no foreseeable reason. The most conscientious and well-supported athletes wind up with injuries, so why should we be any different? Injuries happen.

I don't say this to be discouraging — we can strive to reduce the frequency, intensity, and duration of injury. I'm just saying to *give yourself a break*. Don't see every injury as a rebuke to your style or your habits, just like you shouldn't see every negative review from a client as a soul-rending indictment of your career. Instead, learn what there is to be learned, accept that some things are out of your control, and keep putting one foot in front of the other.

As you do so, I invite you to offer that same grace to your clients. They'll come in with a neck crick and say, "I must have slept wrong" or "I must need a new pillow." Maybe! But sometimes these things just happen, and you don't need to stigmatize the act of sleeping.

I once had a client who had stopped running entirely because of some lateral hip pain she had developed. She had begun to worry that it was a tendon problem and that any further running could set her up for serious injury down the road. Imagine her relief when I told her that, "This is pretty common in runners at your level. I think we'll be able to handle it with some massage and stretching." As our sessions and her training continued, I was able to help her see each little ache as less catastrophic, and more as part of the process. She was glad that she hadn't given up on running, and so was I.

There are so many opportunities in our life to retreat from pain and create a smaller box of what is acceptable and what is healthy. I encourage you to press against that box and keep exploring. Keep playing, experimenting, and dancing.

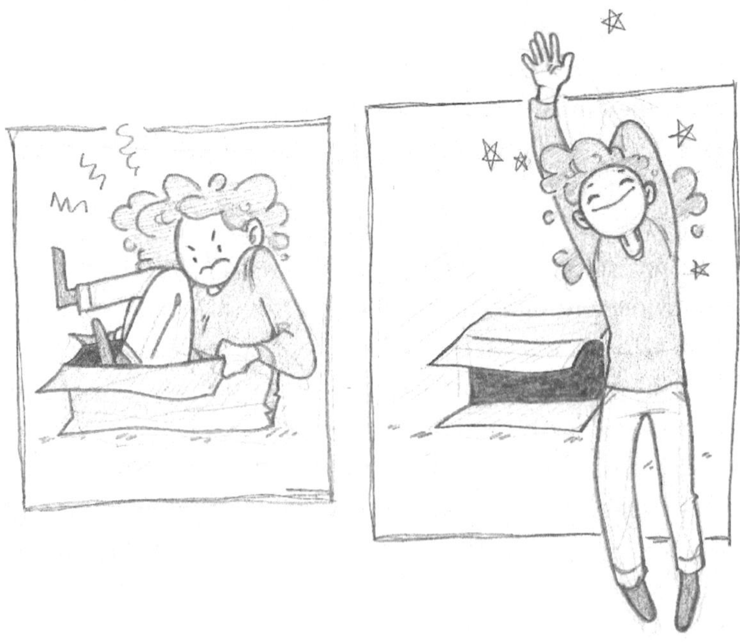

Chapter 6: My Clients Are Driving Me Crazy

There's a common sentiment in the massage universe, and it goes a little something like this: "I wish I never had to see this client again. I always take their energy and end up with a headache, or a bad mood that I can't shake." It can go even further: "I end up taking their back pain and it puts me out of commission for the rest of the day." I was taught by a well-meaning mentor how to shield myself from these negative vibes, using visualization (and my own energy) to protect myself.

It's at this point that I'd like to define the term *meme*. While the internet mostly uses it to describe images and phrases that spread like wildfire, it was originally defined as an idea that's transmitted like a virus. That is, a belief or philosophy that springs up and spreads through populations as if it had gone airborne, often with no clear source and the same exponential growth.

We'll talk about some other massage memes elsewhere – knots, toxins, "it has to hurt for it to work." This idea that we can *take* our client's bad energy, or be directly affected by their pain, follows the same pattern. It's difficult to say where the idea came from, but it's awfully prevalent, and it's often regarded as self-evidently true by its proponents. After all: I made contact with her, I felt her bad energy, and I felt worse afterward.

Like the other memes I mentioned, it's also incorrect. From the last century of psychological studies we've learned a lot about the *psychosomatic effect*, and how we're able to generate very real sensations that seem to be based in our own bodies from nothing but ideas and perceptions. Whether it's seeing a glowing red light and perceiving a probe as "hot," or feeling a poke in a prosthetic hand, the literature on psychogenic pain is very rich[7].

---

[7] https://pubmed.ncbi.nlm.nih.gov/26588692/

We also know quite a bit about empathy, and there's nothing mystical about it. We don't need any sort of energy transmission to explain it, no matter how powerfully we feel it. Humans are social creatures, and we're wired to share experiences, even perceiving them as if we were in someone else's place[8]. While a certain amount of empathy is normal, some people can find their internal mirroring experience to be too powerful, intruding on their ability to live their lives.

It's a fine thing to be empathetic, and it's normal to feel anguish (or even physical pain) when you see someone else hurting, but it can be overwhelming. We don't need energy to explain it. In fact, using the "it's just their bad energy" excuse can lead to some nasty implied finger-pointing.

That client ruined my day.

No, only you can ruin your day. I know, that's something that an annoying uncle would say (coincidentally, I am an uncle, and I'm often annoying), but it's the truth. As much as other people might try to bring us down or stand in our way, we always have power over our internal environment. We can choose how to react, and what perspective to take.

On my first day of massage school, the teachers sat us in a circle and talked with us about communication. See, we were going to be shoved into a pressure cooker with about 20 other students for the next 8 months, and things had a history of getting... testy. The main guideline that they taught us was the use of *I language*.

Instead of saying that someone else did this or that, or that someone else made us feel a certain way, we were encouraged to reframe it using our personal experience:

- Instead of "you hurt my feelings," they wanted us to try, "I'm feeling hurt."
- Instead of "you said that," we'd start with "I heard this."

---

[8] https://pubmed.ncbi.nlm.nih.gov/25893437/

- Instead of speculating on someone else's motivations ("you were trying to upset me"), we'd share what we *imagined* the other party was going through.

It ended up sounding something like this: "I heard you say that I was going to fail the test, and I felt like you were making fun of me. I imagine that you were trying to make a joke, but I'm feeling hurt."

You did this to me!

So, why frame sentences with I language? For one thing, it takes the *accusation* out of the sentence. Even if you're just saying, "you said that...", it can get the listener's back up, making them feel like they've got to play defense. When we're on the defensive, we tend to engage in some bad behavior – name-calling, yelling, and even throwing out some accusations of our own. "Yeah, but *you* said...!"

More importantly, using I language is much truer to the nature of reality. When I say, "I perceive" and "I imagine," I'm admitting that I'm not a perfect witness with perfect recall. I've got a few sensory organs that can record a noisy approximation of a scene, and then I've got a big data processor that tries to recreate it, along with a lot of assumptions and emotions and history thrown in for flavor. When I say that, "you treated me like an idiot," I'm really saying, "my reconstruction of events makes you look like a jerk. Now, defend yourself!"

You may find that shifting the perspective from "you" to "me" also takes some of the anger and fear out of the situation. It lets you sit back and ponder the question, "what am I feeling?" instead of shooting those feelings out of your eyes like laser beams. Interestingly, sitting back and pondering your internal environment can reduce the *intensity* of those feelings. They're still there, but suddenly they seem less powerful, and less immediate. This can make conversations that would usually end in fisticuffs end, hopefully, in tea and hugs.

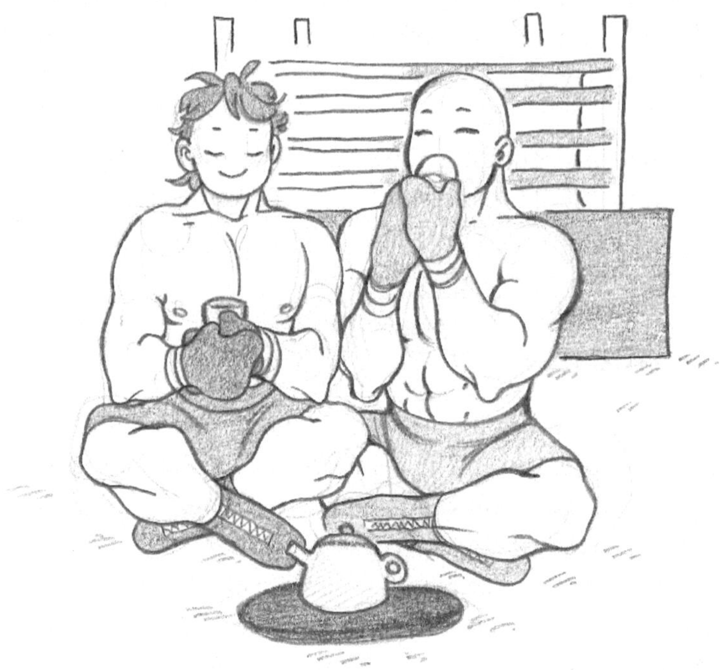

Re: Your client's energy

In psychology, there's this concept called the *locus of control* ("locus" just means "location"). If you perceive yourself having control over a social situation and your reactions to it, you're likely to have better outcomes, and to walk away feeling less angry when things go awry. If you have a deep-down belief that *other people* can ruin your day, your day is way more ruinable.

And so it is with energy. I used to think that my mood and my energy were subject to attacks from the outside. By opening myself to another person, I'd be making myself vulnerable to energy vampires who would leave me psychically beat up and wrung out. My only recourse was to use elaborate grounding strategies and visualizations. While these helped in the moment, and often made my room smell like delicious sage, they were all feeding into my misperception of the locus of control.

How did I stop feeling so tossed about by the seas of temperamental clients and unpredictable social situations? I started by using self-focused language. "What is my experience? Well, I worked on that client, and now I'm exhausted and a little ticked off." Then I looked at my objective experience of their actions, and how I reacted: "Jim didn't speak a lot or make much eye contact. I imagine that he was unhappy to be there. I felt unappreciated." Or, "Jane told me how much her back pain has been affecting her life, and I noticed her shifting repeatedly during the massage. I imagine that she was uncomfortable. I began to feel frustrated by my perceived inability to help her."

All of this analysis and reframing is a pain in the butt at first, but taking that step back and owning your own feelings can help you with the next step: Giving up on mind-reading. Maybe my imagination was correct and Jim didn't appreciate what I was offering as a massage therapist... or maybe Jim was caught up in his own thoughts that day and didn't have much extraversion to spare. Maybe Jane found the entire massage unbearable... or maybe it was a great experience for her, one that she found useful for managing her pain.

Now, the easiest way of figuring out the reality of the situation would be to stick to the facts. Did Jim schedule his next appointment with you? Did Jane report any improvement afterward? Trying to figure out reality is great, but I prefer this option, which we discussed in chapter 1: Giving up on outcomes. Jim liked it, or he didn't. Jane will get better, or she won't. Either way, I gave my best massage possible.

This might sound crazy for a caring profession, but it's worthwhile to recognize that we're not your typical healthcare provider. We're not offering a pill and seeing whether their cholesterol drops. We're not measuring their range of motion with a goniometer and charting their progress over time. Instead, we're dealing with whole humans, usually with several pain complaints and twice as many wellness goals. We provide a complex, meaningful, often intuitive – even artistic – form of systematic contact. While there might be outcomes that we want to track, there's no "wellnessometer."

When I think of our closest relatives in the healthcare community, I don't think of physical therapists or chiropractors. I think of talk therapists, like psychologists and mental health counselors. They spend hour-long sessions with patients. They enter into intimate therapeutic relationships with people who are in pain. And, like us, they rarely get a black-and-white "better" or "worse" verdict after any given session. Like us, they often affect *many* aspects of their patients' lives, not just their mental state.

Talk therapists are taught to distance themselves from the outcome and focus on the process. They're taught to own their own feelings so that it doesn't affect their work, or their home lives. They're told about muddy, weird relationships that can develop with their patients and how to deal with them. As massage therapists, we usually aren't.

Boundaries: The difference between you and me

I want to talk about healthy boundaries and the many benefits these create, but first I'd like to talk about what a complete *lack* of boundaries looks like. Psychologists have a term called *enmeshment*, which means that two or more people are crisscrossed together so thoroughly that it's hard to pick them apart.

In a relationship with terrible boundaries and high enmeshment, you can expect the following dynamics:

- **"Look what you made me do."** Enmeshed couples lose their sense of *agency,* which means the feeling of control over your own actions. This leads to ugly ideas like "you made me lash out," and to equally tragic ideas like...
- **"You make me feel..."** so happy. So sad. So angry.
- **Dependence** and **codependence.** This isn't just *need*, it's *grasping*. It's using someone else as the source of your happiness and fulfillment.

- **Controlling behavior**. Gradual narrowing of a partner's autonomy: "Don't you think you're going out with your friends too often? I'm just worried you'll be tired tomorrow."
- **Transference**. This is where you feel emotions toward someone, whether anger or hatred or love or lust, based on them subconsciously standing in for someone from your past.

All together, these form a sort of relationship "mud." It's sticky, it's gross, it gets on everything, and it acts as a glue that can almost simulate love.

A *boundary* is a statement of values that you use to establish how you and I can safely and happily become *us*. Here are the values that I bring into a relationship:

- I am my own person, both when we're apart and when we're together.
- I am worthy of respect and kindness.
- My body is my own, and I choose when and how I share it.
- My mind is my own. My emotions are mine, and yours are yours.

Once you've got your values in mind, the next step is to translate them into something that can be acted on. Not necessarily strict rules that mean "one strike and you're out" (though there may be breaches that require that), but rather "these are my expectations in a healthy relationship, based on my values, and I ask that they be honored."

How can you communicate these concepts so that they won't be a surprise to a partner, and so that they can feel comfortable sharing their own? If a boundary is crossed, what comes next? This can mean communication (e.g., "I heard you say this, and I felt disrespected."), compromise (e.g., if a partner feels unsafe when you drink, your bodily autonomy doesn't trump their need for safety; you might offer to abstain), or consequences, up to and including separation.

What are your lines in the sand? What can be solved by communication, and what represents an unacceptable breach of your boundaries?

Boundaries in a therapeutic relationship

If you're a new massage therapist or student, I'm going to warn you right now: It's not as simple as it sounded in your business ethics class. You'll forge strong bonds with some clients over the months and years of working closely with them. They'll find an escape from pain and new body awareness that will be just as awe-inspiring for you as it is for them. Some clients will have whole entire babies while under your care, they'll change careers, and some will move away and move back for a joyous reunion. Sometimes you'll accompany a client, one you've known for years, along that last journey from sickness, to dying, to death.

That entire time, you'll be living your life as well. Maybe you'll move to a new workplace and find that lots of clients follow you. These will be your true-blue supporters and cheerleaders, and the ones who are still there five years later will be counted among your oldest friends. You'll have long conversations with some of them, spanning many sessions and skipping across long silences like a flat stone on a still pond. They'll share your joy when you have successes and offer comfort when you're feeling low.

Overcoming pain together. Exploring the body together. Spending long stretches of silence together. These are the everyday realities for a massage therapist and their client, and they can represent fertile ground for a relationship to form. You have a few options for how to deal with this near inevitability:

1. **Staunch rejection**. This is the approach to setting boundaries that seems to be favored by armchair ethicists on internet forums (be careful where you get your ethics, folks). It requires you to be a perfect conduit for healthcare and nothing else. Small talk is forbidden, unless it's about fascia!

2. **Entanglement**. Whatever happens, happens. If you hit it off with a client, why not divulge a few secrets and talk about past relationships with them? Why not have lunch or set up a playdate between your kids? You can set boundaries later, after resentment sets in!
3. **Mindful growth**. Allowing rapport to grow, and even friendship to develop, while keeping an eye toward your values as a massage therapist.

Think of this last path as a trellis meant to guide the growth of relationships in the context of therapeutic goals. That's the *therapeutic relationship* that you may have heard me talk about: A mutually supportive and open rapport between therapist and client, with the ultimate goal of facilitating clinical outcomes. This is the context that allows a client to feel safe enough to discuss their sacrum pain, which they'd never brought up with other practitioners. It's a place where you can find your voice and communicate difficult concepts, allowing you to try new approaches with informed consent. It's a relationship that allows your massage office to feel like a haven from the outside world, one with healing properties of its own.

There will still be some chaos inherent to the process, but it can be dealt with and guided if you keep your professional boundaries in mind. Start with general statements of your values, and then translate those to actionable guidelines. I'll tell you mine, but yours don't have to be exactly the same, or stated in the same way:

- My time and expertise are worth money.
- My mental health and personal life are more important than money.
- I am a trained professional worthy of respect. I am not a machine.
- My practice is client-focused, and my client is the expert on their own body.
- My practice is full-human focused.
- I acknowledge the power differential in my treatment room.
- The burden of effective communication falls on me.

- Both my client and I maintain our bodily autonomy at all times.
- My emotions are my own. My client's emotions are their own.

These are ideas that took years to develop, and I'm still in the process of implementing them. You won't have a perfect practice at first, or perfect boundaries. Just realize that by having your values in mind, you'll find that you can set goals for how you'd like to be treated, and how you'd like to offer work.

I am not a machine. That means I acknowledge that my body is biological and capable of being overburdened. I don't need to acquiesce to every demand for more pressure, or give in when a boss asks me to work longer shifts. I'm a human being, darn it, and humans need rest! As a trained professional worthy of respect, I'm the expert in the room when it comes to my limits, or whether massage is contraindicated.

My time is worth money, and my mental health is priceless. For me, that means mostly eliminating discounts and freebies, as well as being strict about when I'm willing to offer sessions. I don't let people schedule same-day appointments (even if I'm already at the office!), or pack extra sessions onto the end of a long day. Yes, I'm leaving money on the table, and yes, my mental health is worth it.

I acknowledge the power differential in the client-therapist relationship, and my practice is client-focused. Realizing this has a lot of implications.

Acknowledging your power

Being someone's massage therapist involves a *power differential*. This means that you seem powerful, and your client might feel powerless in comparison. Consider this: They come to you, an expert, often with a problem that's difficult to describe. They're expected to divulge their own medical history, sometimes in excruciating detail on rather invasive intake forms, and then to remove their clothes, often with minimal instruction. Then they lie face down, passive and naked and maybe a little cold, and wait for this near-stranger to walk in and place their hands on their body. Once the massage begins, are they allowed to ask for more pressure? Are they allowed to speak up if it hurts? Are they allowed to leave if they don't like it?

That's how intimidating and powerless being a client *can* feel, but it doesn't have to be that way. I believe that our number one job as massage therapists, above anatomy knowledge or manual therapy skills, is to mitigate that power imbalance and help the client realize that they are in control, and that they are the expert when it comes to the deep and intricate topic of their unique body.

Imagine this: You walk into a massage therapist's office for the first time, but you already feel like you know it. You've seen pictures and you know what to expect. Your massage therapist walks in, and you feel like you know them! They've spent a lot of time answering questions on their website or social media, and maybe they've even posted some videos (more on this later). They shake your hand warmly, welcome you back to the massage room, and ask you to have a seat. They sit on a stool so that they're looking up at you rather than looming over you. They let you talk as much as you need to, genuinely interested in how your body works and what's worked for you in the past, and then they explain the upcoming session. They invite you to speak up if you experience anything interesting or related to your pain. They ask you not to suffer in silence, and tell you that you're in control of the session. They talk about how much to undress, how to lie on the table, and when to expect a knock on the door. When they reenter the room, they place their hands gently and slowly, making it seem like a question rather than a statement.

When I think of the best massages I've ever received, I think of ones where I felt ease and comfort, and where the massage was truly tailored to me. When I think of the worst, I think of ones where I felt like sheet metal in a factory, rushed through and smashed into a predetermined shape.

Empowering the client is good ethics, and it's good massage therapy. Clients who feel more in control will be more open about their goals and their experiences on the table, and they'll feel a stronger connection to the work. They'll feel like a partner rather than an object, a co-creator in their own wellness.

Just realize that the power differential will always exist to some extent, no matter how you try to create balance. Even as friendships develop and conversations are shared, and even as years pass, I ask that you remember that you are still the therapist, and they are still the client. You are still applying while they are receiving. Boundaries might get muddy here and there as relationships transform, but remember where things started, and that being client-focused means knowing when and where to step back, or to step on the brakes. See the interlude following this chapter for more.

My emotions are mine, and yours are yours

Earlier in this chapter, I said that we don't need energy to explain the feeling of "taking" someone's bad mood or bad back. But suppose I'm off the mark there, and there is an invisible interplay of energy between humans, doing work behind the scenes. Maybe electromagnetic, or spiritual, or divine. There are plenty of strange and wondrous phenomena in the universe, and I'd be happy to be wrong.

Even in the case of energy passing between me and my client, I can still claim my own space. I can still choose to own my emotions and guide my resulting actions. If a client consistently leaves me in a bad mood, I can dig deeper to try to figure out where that's coming from, and see if there's a change I need to make.

Just realize that the earlier you choose who you want to be as a professional, and the earlier you start creating your workplace's culture, the harder it is to wind up with lots of client-related stress or co-worker-related stress. Choose how you're willing to be treated, recognize boundary-pushing early and treat it early, and you'll find that your days in this industry can be pleasantly serene.

Interlude: Transference, Relationships, and Misconduct

So, you've set your boundaries, you've created a culture of safety and client-focused care, and yet...

You've hit it off with someone. A client. You think you might be in love. Or in lust. Or they're pursuing you and you don't quite feel it but you consider them a friend, and you can't just fire them! But should you? Or what if it's mutual and you want to forget the whole massage thing and try dating?

As you consider whether to expand or disband the client-therapist relationship, be aware of *transference*. This is the phenomenon where we unconsciously use people in our lives as stand-ins for past relationships, be they familial or romantic or otherwise. Some clients get swept away by the quality of nonjudgmental care that massage therapists provide, and their minds can start viewing us through the filter of "lover" or "parent." This can masquerade as love or connection, but this person isn't seeing *you*, they're seeing a parent who isn't absent, or an old lover who is physically caring. They might also see an old enemy, or a former abuser.

Transference can happen in the other direction too. This can happen silently during sessions or based on conversations, but you might find yourself infatuated with a client. You look forward to their sessions and find their approval very important, and you wonder if they feel the same about you and... darn it, that's not your client, that's someone else! You've taken this person and slotted them into a template in your brain that represents an old connection you had, or an old trauma, or both. And all while this person is just trying to get their wonky left shoulder back into gear.

I bring up these phenomena because they're likely to occur in a therapeutic context, and because they can *feel* authentic and organic. If one member of a therapeutic relationship becomes infatuated with the other, it can feel like a real connection, and it can feel potent. It can even be reciprocated! But this is the part where massage therapists need to be the professional in the room and remember to put the client and their mental and physical health above all else. Be aware that transference can interfere with the healing process because it can lead clients to be overly submissive, or resistant to treatment, neither of which is optimal when you're trying to do collaborative work. It can lead a therapist to set good therapy aside in pursuit of their infatuation.

This can also be the source of the "bad energy" that we talked about earlier. It might feel like this person has bad mojo, but the source is something from your past that hasn't been fully worked out. Against all odds, this 30-year-old college administrator might be reminding you of your childhood relationship with your dad. The brain is weird in ways that should never be underestimated.

So, what to do about social messiness and psychological weirdness in the context of massage? Be aware of it, remember your boundaries, and keep your focus on a balanced therapeutic relationship. Just by acknowledging the possibility of transference to yourself and choosing not to get swept away in these misplaced feelings, you can rob them of most of their momentum.

Be willing to have difficult conversations. If a client clearly has a raging crush and it's leading to inappropriate behavior, or if the client is needlessly rude and is treating you poorly, it's the massage therapist's responsibility to say, "Could we have a quick chat? I've got some concerns I'd like to talk about." Say those words, keep your values in mind, and let the rest of the conversation take care of itself. If you'd like to game out the next step, it might sound something like this: "I've noticed this, and I'm feeling..." That's right, self-focused language!

Be willing to put a stop to a relationship that crosses boundaries. If a client is writing you poetry and gazing into your eyes as you work, or if you find yourself obsessing over someone who just wants to relax, it can reach the point where the massage therapist needs to make the decision to step away. Consider an email that says, "Joe, I feel the need to draw our work together to a close. This is for personal reasons and isn't a reflection on you. There's another massage therapist I'd like you to try who I think will be an excellent fit. Please let me know if you have any questions." If the client doesn't intuit the reasoning and asks for an explanation, you can always go with, "I'm having some emotional stuff that comes up during our sessions. Again, it's nothing to do with you, but it's something I need to resolve on my own. Thanks for understanding, and I wish you the best."

But what if it's not transference?

That happens, and like I said before, therapeutic relationships can readily morph into friendships. Even if you've got your professional values firmly in hand and you're keeping an eye out for transference and other types of enmeshment, sometimes you might find that you and a client really click. If the two of you had met in a class or a club, you'd be exchanging social media handles on day one and watching anime marathons by day three.

This is when I ask that you be mindful of the *dual relationship* phenomenon. A dual or multiple relationship is one where you try to be someone's massage therapist *and* their friend. Their girlfriend and their co-worker. Their doctor and their business partner. I'm not asking you to rule out such complex arrangements completely, just to recognize that they can have inherent logistical problems, and that they can be messy.

Let's say you have a client who is a fellow runner, and after twenty sessions she invites you to train with her and her marathon group. That's a dual relationship, and possibly a step into a deeper friendship... but that feels pretty safe to me. Sturdy, as far as such things go. If you notice that particular client taking liberties with your time by suddenly canceling more often or showing up late and expecting her full time, you can still communicate firmer boundaries without either of those two relationships being mortally wounded.

But let's say that a client asks you on a date, and there does seem to be a straightforward connection. Can you go on that date and keep that person as your client? Can you turn down that date and keep that person as your client?

To put it simply: No, and maybe not. Romance and romantic interest, especially in their initial stages, are just thematically incompatible with a therapeutic relationship. The client's feeling of safety might be compromised, as can their feeling of bodily autonomy. The power differential could be thrown completely out of balance, and the expression of yourself as a professional could be undermined.

I don't have any hard rules for you here, like requiring that you space a massage relationship and a romantic relationship out by 6 months. I don't expect you to fire every client who seems to have a bit of a crush. I just want you to be aware of your responsibility to your clients to do no harm, and I also want you to make your own life easier. If you enter into a dual relationship of any sort, do so with your eyes open and a plan for what to do if things go sour.

If you do choose to stop seeing someone as a client to focus on another form of relationship, I ask that you remember where you came from. They were originally your client, and you were originally their therapist. Keep an eye out for aftereffects of that, especially if your new friend/girlfriend/boss/student treats you with deference. There might still be a power differential, and that could require communication to gradually uproot.

On sexual misconduct

If you follow "massage" as a topic on any news app, there's a frequent and recurring theme to the articles: Clients being preyed upon and abused in a massage office. Sometimes there's a new story every day about a massage therapist, fully licensed and working under the auspices of a professional organization, facing accusations about inappropriate and unwanted sexual contact. I imagine that the numbers are larger than this, because posts on massage therapy forums are frequently titled something like, "should I report him?" or, "was this inappropriate?" In other words, there is a sexual assault problem in the field of massage therapy, we're not doing anything concerted to counter it, and it makes me feel like I'm going crazy.

A common refrain in feminist thought is, "instead of teaching women how to avoid rape, teach men not to rape." And that's exactly what I'd like us to do. Because I feel convinced that very few men enter this field with the intention of harming clients. The vast majority join up because they've enjoyed massage in the past, and they'd like to help people in the same way. They make it all the way through massage school, with all the new anatomy and kinesiology knowledge, and great information about all sorts of musculoskeletal injuries and conditions. They spend years applying this knowledge, forging therapeutic relationships and helping people out of pain. And then, one day, maybe a decade later, their mugshot is on the local news sites and the afternoon news hour.

Here's what I imagine happens: Rather than these men starting out as wolves in sheep's clothing, their descent into misconduct takes time, and it involves a gradual corruption of their professional ethics and boundaries. Maybe they were never taught about the power differential, or the importance of robust consent to a therapeutic relationship. As they find themselves infatuated with certain clients, they're not familiar enough with the concept of transference to instantly and emphatically step back. I'm not saying this to exonerate these men — I'm saying that maybe, with the proper education and forewarning, great harm could be prevented. Rather than wandering blithely into infatuation and letting it interact with their libido, a man who is forewarned and forearmed might say, "I remember this from massage school, and I don't want to do anything without consent." I believe that evil is a process, and it can be interrupted.

So, massage schools and massage teachers, please take a look at your ethics class. Is there a point in which you talk about the sexual assault epidemic at massage franchises that was widely reported in the 2010s? Is there a section on mindfulness and how unethical behavior can slowly creep in? Do you warn them against the practice of rationalizing misconduct, and how that can be a self-perpetuating process? How much of your emphasis is on robust consent and balancing the power differential?

Because if your ethics class consists mostly of "don't date clients" (in other words, abstinence education), then you're setting your students up to fail. Email me. Let's talk about the psychology of corruption, the seductive qualities of power, and the slow creep of evil. We'll chart out a two-week lesson plan.

Chapter 7: Business Is Scary!

If you're a new massage therapist, the thought of going into business for yourself can be intimidating. Quarterly taxes, bookkeeping, licenses, inspections, local and state laws, finding and keeping clients. It all seems like so much! Surely you need to work for someone else for ten years and let them take 75% of your income before you even think about it!

But I've got good news from the future: You eventually took all those steps, and they were all *easy*. Like, astoundingly easy, and once you did them you were left wondering what you were so worried about in the first place.

Let's start with a basic truth about business, whether massage-related or not: A million people have already walked the exact route that you plan to walk, and every well-trodden path gets paved. What currently feels like a scary unknown world to you is actually fully mapped out, with whole government agencies and private industries set up just to usher you to the business of your dreams.

Navigating laws and taxes

The most cumbersome part of this process is figuring out the local requirements for setting up shop. Here in the U.S., that means figuring out what your city requires, what your county requires, and what your state requires. I've lived in places where each of these entities wanted a piece of the pie (meaning a business license with a fee every two years), which was in stark contrast to another state I worked in where nobody seemed to care if I rented an office and called it a business. Frankly, I prefer when everyone wants money. It makes me less suspicious.

The easiest way to navigate this process in the U.S. is to take advantage of your local small business development center (SBDC). These are government-sponsored groups of business consultants who want nothing more than to get your small business off the ground!

Just search "[my city] SBDC" to find one near you and see what information they have online. That might be enough to get you going; if not, make a free appointment for a consultation, and a nice business major or accountant will walk you through every little thing.

Other useful resources:

- Local massage therapist message boards, which are easiest to find on Facebook. If one exists for your area, you'll likely find that many threads about how to start a business already exist. Just make sure to double-check any information that isn't backed up with sources.
- The local chapter of a regional massage group, such as the American Massage Therapy Association (AMTA). Chances are there's one in your area. You can attend a meeting, or just shoot them a call or message with questions.
- Your state's massage licensure board. Some of these are more helpful than others – your state board might have all the information you need on their website with responsive staff to answer questions, or you might find what looks like an old GeoCities page and no good way to get a response from a human.

Here's what the process looks like in my area of Florida: Get a business license from the city and from the county, both of which need to be done in person for some reason. There are some boxes to check and a small fee to pay, and then you get a piece of paper to display in your office. Once you've got that office, you need an inspection from the state board, which you set up in advance. They make sure you have clean facilities and necessary safety equipment like a fire extinguisher and soap, and then you're ready to start seeing clients!

There's also the small matter of paying taxes. This is easy when you're working for someone as an employee: They handle the withholding, they pay extra tax for the privilege of being an employer, and they give you a piece of paper (your W-2) with all the relevant numbers at the end of the year.

When you employ yourself or act as a contractor, the federal government expects quarterly tax payments, and your state might as well. You have to keep track of all your income, as well as all your business expenses, and then show your work on a form when you file your yearly taxes (this is called the Schedule C). **I know this sounds scary**, I really do, but once you've done it a single time, you'll wonder what you were scared of.

Tracking your income and expenses can be incredibly easy. You can do it by hand in a spreadsheet or notebook, or you can use an app. I use one called "QuickBooks Self-Employed" that costs about 20 bucks a month. It digests all the information from my bank account, I tell it which bits are me making money and which bits are me spending money on my business, and over time you train it to pretty much do all the work itself. For instance, it knows that all my Taco Bell spending is personal and should be excluded from the calculations, so it doesn't even bother me about those costs. It doesn't judge me either, which I appreciate.

As you make money, it will calculate your estimated quarterly taxes, which you pay via an IRS website. At the end of the year, you can use the data collected by your app to fill in all the relevant numbers in your tax software, or you can hire a CPA (certified public accountant) and give them access to that info so that they can do all the number juggling and make sure you didn't miss any deductions. Again: Sounds scary, but you'll be surprised by how easy it is once you've done it.

What about LLCs and EINs and DBAs?!

Oh my. Here's where I'm going to say something that will sound like blasphemy to internet forum business experts: You don't gotta worry about forming a limited liability corporation (LLC) at first. Just by opening up shop and doing business, you're automatically a business type called a "sole proprietorship," which means that *you are* the business. When the business makes money, you make money. All your finances are one and the same, and it makes doing taxes at the end of the year a fairly frictionless process.

"But Ian! LLCs protect your personal assets if you're sued!" Sometimes! But your professional liability insurance is much more likely to do the heavy lifting there. In some cases you'll be able to rent commercial real estate via your LLC, but for a single massage therapist looking for a small office, they're likely to require a personal guarantee. That's how landlords sidestep LLCs entirely, leaving you on the hook if you need to default on a lease. LLCs aren't foolproof, they're not your first line of defense, and they can usually wait until you get your feet under you.

You can choose to get an EIN, an employer identification number, for free through the IRS website. This lets you use that number instead of your social security number for things like issuing 1099 forms, applying for business licenses, opening a business banking account, and filing your taxes. It can be nice to not throw your SSN around to everyone who wants a number on a form.

If you want to call your business something other than your own name, you'll need to file a DBA ("doing business as") form with your state. So, if you want to be "Blooming Chrysanthemum Day Spa," which I think sounds very pretty, but also like a dish at Outback Steakhouse, you'll need to search for how to register that name in your particular location. For this and everything else above, your local small business development center will be your best resource.

Getting off the ground

My advice here is to start with what's easy and expand as needed. Start as a sole proprietor, get yourself some accounting software, and keep track of your expenses as you start up. You can deduct every penny you spend on rent, utilities, supplies (keep or scan your receipts!), licensing fees, and whatever software and apps you use to support your business. There are lots of other deductions as well, so take some time to do a little research every time you ask yourself, "hmm, is this business-related or personal?" If it's necessary to keep your business running, chances are that you can deduct it.

The next step is to find an office, or to be a mobile massage therapist, or both. This part can seem intimidating, but the easiest way is to find a local massage therapist who isn't using their room for several days a week and pay them to use it on those off days. It's cheaper than getting your own room, and it takes care of pesky issues like finding furniture. In some states you can even piggyback on their establishment license and not need to go through that process at all!

Many massage therapists will also have extra rooms for rent or for sharing. Be cautious when pursuing this route — look for pure rental situations rather than messy "you work for me, I make all the rules, but there's no contract and you're not my employee" arrangements. Even in more structured situations like working out of a spa or clinic, you'll often find that they expect to take the lion's share of income when you're the one doing the actual work. Doesn't make sense to me, no matter how many times business owners talk down to me about it.

Instead, how about a nice office all your own? There are office complexes in just about every city, often in great abundance, that will provide you with a 12'x12' room for a few hundred bucks per month. You put your sign up on the door, they might put a sign up for you outside the complex, and there's usually a communal waiting room that your clients can sit in. In order to find these, you can search the internet for "office space in [my city]" and search listings, or reach out directly to commercial real estate agents. The latter is much more likely to bear fruit, especially in cities that aren't very online. They'll know all the nooks and crannies where those single rooms exist.

As you search, realize that you don't have to take a bum deal. Some realtors will want you to sign a two-year lease with no exit clause, which is an utterly mad proposition for someone just getting their feet wet. Ask for shorter contracts and see what they're willing to offer; if they won't negotiate to make things more newbie friendly, thank them for their time and keep asking around.

But what about clients?!

Oh, that's the easy part. The trick here is to disregard every bit of conventional wisdom about finding clients and listen to me instead.

... I'm only half joking there. The conventional wisdom around finding new clients for any profession sounds something like this: Join a business networking group where you pay a fee to make monthly sales pitches to other local business owners who have also paid a fee. Go door to door, pounding the pavement and spreading news of your business far and wide to other businesses. Buy a billboard. Buy an ad in the yellow pages(?!). Donate gift certificates to charity. Give away chair massage on a regular basis. Deeply discount your sessions, either through a service like Groupon or on your own. Give away a hundred gift certificates and upsell as hard as you can when those clients arrive.

And some of these can be effective, if managed correctly and using the right strategies. Free chair massage can turn into paid clients *if* you're able to sell your services during the treatment and sign them up for a table massage right after. Groupon can work *if* you limit the number and recognize that you need to have an extra hook to appeal to bargain-hunting massage tourists. Pounding the pavement can work *if* you target a certain niche of businesses and appeal to them specifically (more on this in a moment).

Basically, the conventional wisdom has you either casting an overly broad net and likely wasting money on low-return strategies (e.g., buying ad space in the newspaper), or discounting your own time deeply and relying on excellent sales skills to convert cheap service to lucrative service. Make no mistake, when someone says, "giving away chair massage works for me," they usually mean, "I really know how to close a sale." An excellent skill to have and cultivate, but not necessarily something that a new massage therapist can access on day one. Trying to figure it out on the fly could lead to a lot of frustration, all while creating a perception of low value for your business.

Instead, why not appeal to the exact people that you're looking for as clients? If you love working with athletes, why not give a nudge to every athlete within five miles of your business, maybe beaming a video of yourself giving a beautiful sports massage directly to their phone? I am, of course, talking about online advertising.

Online ads: Not just for mattresses and workout gear

I've had to start over a few times in my massage career, suddenly needing to find all new clients in an unfamiliar area. I had no inroads to get word-of-mouth started, and I didn't even know the local area all that well. Fortunately, every major social media platform knows every person in your city better than they know themselves, and the panopticon is willing to show them your ads for mere pennies per exposure!

This is something that works for every platform, whether it be Facebook or Google or Instagram: Make something attention-grabbing, add a little info, and then start serving that as an ad to people in your area who might be interested in your work. Dump a hundred dollars into it every month, tweak it as you figure out what gets the best responses, and then slowly taper off advertising as your schedule fills up.

This is something worth researching so that you know the best practices and the right options to select for each platform, but as always, I advise you to get the ball rolling, and *then* figure out all the little details. Make a Facebook business page and start boosting it to your local area. You can boost the page itself or individual posts, or a combination of both. Play around with it, and realize that no single exposure is likely to get you a new client. This is a matter of people seeing your name ten times over the course of a few months and thinking, "hmm, maybe I should give them a try."

As for who to target, think about your ideal client. I love working with nurses, triathletes, and office workers. If a yoga or Pilates practitioner finds their way into my office, I'm pleased as punch. I love working with CrossFitters because they're always down for some active engagement. Because I'm not exactly picky, it would be easy for me to cast too wide a net and end up not appealing to anyone! Instead, narrow the groups that you're targeting, and try to put yourself in their shoes. What would grab their attention as they scroll down their Facebook or Instagram feed? Again, this is something that you can tinker with as you move forward, so don't feel like you're locked into any one strategy.

Before we move on, let me tell you about the most effective ad I've ever seen. I was scrolling Instagram, liking people's food pics, art, and massage studio setups, and suddenly a video said, "Hey y'all, this is Engine Guy. Need to get your car fixed? Call Engine Guy! We do spark plugs, we do brakes, we do engines. Find us on Google, five-star reviews! Check us out on our website. Thanks, and I hope to see you here." It was literally a guy in his shop talking into his selfie cam, and I've never felt such a powerful connection with a stranger. Just a guy being himself, being awkwardly enthusiastic, leaving in all the pauses and "ums," and just going for it. Be like Engine Guy, and just go for it.

Your informative online presence

All this advertising stuff, and even word of mouth, all works better if you have an informative online presence. By that I mean that potential clients can get to know you before they ever step into your office, and they can have all their questions answered and their fears allayed.

Think about what it's like to look for a massage therapist in a new town. You've got certain characteristics you're looking for (maybe you've got a favorite modality), but you're mostly looking for someone you can trust to be a professional. This is a pricey service, so you want at least some reassurance that this person knows what they're doing and won't waste your time or money. What can you post online that will not only help these people find you when they search, but also make them feel confident enough to press a "book now" button?

First things first: Establish a *broad* online presence, and make it all link together. This lets clients find your business on Facebook, scroll through your pictures and demonstration videos on Instagram, and then look up your reviews on Google maps. They can then spend a few minutes poking around your website, checking your "about me" page, and maybe reading some blog posts. It gives your business a sense of weight – contrast that with the perception of a single page on Facebook, or one whipped up through a free site builder. That can seem rather flimsy, and can leave people wondering whether this business is open (or even real!).

Instead, build yourself a real website with a real web address. This is easy enough using a paid site builder like Squarespace or Wix. It will be a couple hundred dollars per year, but they'll take care of the general look and feel, and they'll handle most of the background optimization needed to get you to show up on search engines (i.e., SEO). Have this link to your Facebook business page and your Google Maps profile, and list your new website on your business social media. Having this interlinking web of sites and profiles is another way that search engines determine that you're legitimate, which makes you more likely to be higher on the list when people search for massage in your area.

Second: Make that broad online presence informative. When people click an ad link that brings them to your Facebook business page, they should be able to immediately see some pictures of your studio (inviting!), read some of your answers to frequently asked client questions (reassuring!), and maybe even see you in action in a video. From there they might click the link to your website. There they'll find more pictures, a list of your services and prices, your cancellation policy and other professional necessities, and... paragraphs! Your website is the best place to spend some time really telling clients about who you are and what you do.

This can be an introduction on the home page, an "about me" page (a great place to put the school you graduated from, any continuing education you've taken, and your general approach to massage), and a blog that you use to answer client questions and allay possible fears. I like to have a blog post that walks people through their first ever session — here's what you'll fill out, here's what the interview will be like, here's what getting on the table will be like, and here's what I'd like to hear from you during the massage. I like to use other blog posts to directly address different client groups, telling athletes about how massage can be a useful part of their training regimen, and telling office workers how we can keep them feeling comfortable in their cubicle. I also like to address specific pain conditions like headache, jaw pain, and fibromyalgia.

As you write these posts, realize that you don't need all the answers. You just need to talk about your clinical experience, your approach to these different scenarios, and what benefits you expect for your clients. Also realize that you can do all the self-plagiarism you like! As you write your blog post, try to find little snippets that you can post along with a picture to Instagram. As you post a picture to Instagram, think about whether it would be a good fit for your Facebook business page (indeed, cross-posting between these two platforms can be set to happen automatically).

Finally: Realize that all this online stuff is a forgiving process, and that there are a hundred "right" ways to do it. You can do well with just a Facebook business page, or just a listing on Yelp. You don't need to write blog posts, and your "about me" page can be a little sparse. All your photos and videos can be taken from your phone. You don't need a logo or a business name, and you can get by without business cards (though people will ask for them, so they're nice to have).

Don't let anyone tell you that there's one right way to present yourself as a business. You can post on your social media ten times per week, or once per month, or forget it exists for months at a time. I find that consistency and thoroughness in my online presence can help, but I've also found that disappearing for a while doesn't particularly hurt me, and that people are enthusiastic when I finally post something new. All this business stuff can be intimidating, all this tech stuff especially so. Start small, start with what's easy and doable, and expand from there.

A quick word on creepers

In chapter 4 we talked about creeper-proofing your practice, and there are some changes that you can make to your online presence to keep them moving along:

1. **No same-day booking**. I'm not exaggerating when I say that this can eliminate 90% of your encounters with ill-intentioned dudes. Make this policy clear on your website, cite it when you get messages or texts from new people who are looking for an appointment that day, and bake it into your online scheduling (any scheduling software worth its salt will have the option to prevent same-day booking). Creeps do not deal well with delayed gratification, and this will get you a higher quality of client in general.
2. **Require information**. Whether you schedule by phone or by an online service, requiring a little information can be all it takes to deter bad actors. Asking for a phone number, email address, and physical address can do the trick. Requiring a credit card number on file can be even better. Just realize that the more hoops that you require a new client to jump through, the more likely you are to deter ideal clients as well (more on this in a moment).
3. **Save your ad money**. If your advertising seems to be drawing in an unusual number of creeps, you can try refining your targeting ("triathletes" can get you a more select group of athletes than "runners," for instance), or you can turn off advertising for men altogether. You'll still get male clients from word of mouth, but these are much more likely to be ideal clients than what you'd get from casting a wide net. Just realize that changing your gender targeting can potentially exclude nonbinary and other gender nonconforming clients, so consider doing extra outreach to make sure that they know that you exist, and that they're welcome on your table.

There are other strategies that might fit with your business, such as featuring prenatal massage prominently in your services and blog posts – this can make ideal clients feel safe, even if they're not looking for prenatal massage, and it can make creepers think twice about whether you're a suitable target. The same can be true for infant massage classes, meditation or yoga workshops, and other nurturing offerings that signal that your business is all about healing and wellness.

You can add explicit language about sexual solicitation on your intake form, with something along the lines of, "by signing below you agree that any form of sexual solicitation, harassment, or other misconduct will result in the immediate termination of the session with full payment due." You can do something similar on your website, clearly and concisely stating that no sexual services are offered, and that solicitation will result in cessation of the session, or contacting the police. Just realize that such language can seem intimidating to well-intentioned clients, and can do little to deter a creeper. In fact, some of them seek out businesses that explicitly disavow sexual services, because they perceive it as a wink and a nod that, yes, actually, sexual services are offered here.

If you'd like to include a disclaimer on your site, I recommend doing so with a link to a long-form post, explaining how massage is distinct and separate from sex. You can talk about client concerns here, such as involuntary arousal, and how they don't need to worry about their autonomic responses and should allow such concerns to float on by. Finally, in this broader context, you can directly address the problem of therapist harassment in this industry, and the damaging effects it can have on morale and your sense of safety. You can ask that clients who are seeking sex do so elsewhere, and set down consequences for stepping over these reasonable boundaries.

As you consider these strategies, just realize that you can't control what people with bad intentions do, and it can be an exercise in frustration to try and organize your business or your life around their inscrutable whims. You can try to make your business invincible to chaos by deleting your headshot, having only a picture of a bare table in an undecorated room, and writing only in the most clinical of terms, but remember that what creepers do isn't about you, it's about them. Yes, project a professional image and take reasonable precautions, but keep your warmth, keep your personality, and draw in your ideal clients until there's simply no room for nonsense.

My secret weapons

The best way to get clients is to put yourself in their shoes, and to do the work that other local massage therapists aren't doing to draw in hesitant or first-time clients. You've started this process already by building up an informative online presence — in a sea of therapists who have somewhat similar single-page profiles, yours will do far more to get clients on board with your massage philosophy. You'll find that people walk into your office already enthusiastic about your approach, and with their questions partly answered. It's like starting a race at the halfway mark and the wind at your back!

We'll discuss a variety of marketing strategies, but let's start with the ones that really make things easy:

Make videos of yourself in action. When it comes to answering questions about who you are and how you work, nothing comes close to the impact of video. Grab a friend to act as camera operator (or use a tripod with a phone mount attachment), bring an extra lamp or two into your treatment room for more light, and ask a trusted friend or client if they'd like to lie on the table while you make promo material. Any phone from the last five years can capture decent video, and there are plenty of paid and free apps that will let you cut it down to size, and even add a bit of narration on top (if you want to be like Engine Guy).

Keep these videos short and punchy. Cutting them down to less than a minute is a good guideline that maximizes compatibility with most social media sites, and it's more likely to keep people's attention for the entire duration. Start with action — the first second should show hands at work — and try to imagine what would prompt you to take a momentary breather as you scroll down an endless feed of vacation pics and latte foam art. Hands gliding down either side of the spine are a thing of beauty, as is the sight of the upper trapezius being plucked up for some petrissage. Showcase your best work, and consider cutting from scene to scene before your viewer's scrolling thumb gets itchy.

From there, you can just post the video! Getting into the habit of putting action videos into the mix, along with pictures of your studio and the great lunch you got at a local eatery and your dog dressed as Chewbacca (business accounts don't have to be strictly business), can be very effective at drawing clients' curiosity and convincing them over time. You can also throw some advertising dollars at them: By boosting a video on Facebook or Instagram, you can ensure that your local hair stylists see your amazing hand and forearm massage video, and that local runners see your sports massage routine.

This is actually my number one strategy for finding new clients, so I want to give it some extra emphasis: By advertising using videos of yourself in action, you are likely to get much more bang for your buck, and to get more clients more quickly. It's great to advertise using photos of yourself and your space, and to get your website in front of people, but a video can make a client say, "man, I really could use a massage. I could use *that* massage."

Make booking easy. Here's something I've experienced in the past: I was looking for a local yoga studio to try out, and I found a likely candidate. Good reviews, nice pictures, and there was a beginner's class coming up. There was no way to book directly from the Facebook page I was looking at, so I went to their website, found the link to their scheduler (it was on the "classes" tab, which took some searching), and gave it a click. I was taken to their introduction page on *another* website which had a different appearance and layout, which meant hunting down my preferred class again. I found it, clicked the "schedule now" link, and was told that I'd need to create an account and sign in before I could proceed. I contemplated my life for a moment, closed the window, and then went to the gym instead.

Compare that to this experience: Whether you're on Facebook, Instagram, or my website, there is *always* an easy-to-find button that says "book now." This takes you to a list of my services (60-minute or 90-minute sessions — I don't want to overwhelm people with choice, and I offer add-ons later in the process), and a quick list of my upcoming openings. Click one of those, enter some information, click a box to agree to my cancellation policy, and you're done. From beginning to end, you can go from curiosity to commitment in about three minutes. My software sends a confirmation email with information on when to arrive, how to find my office, and a reminder of my policies. They get another reminder via email and text the day before their appointment, all without me touching my phone or pressing a button.

The point of all of this: Think about accessibility as it relates to getting clients on your schedule, and as it relates to making your own life easier. Every extra click, every unfamiliar screen that requires a mental reorientation, and every hoop to jump through (like asking people to sign up for yet another website) is an off-ramp from your corner of the internet. Marketers call this "bounce rate," and nothing causes people to bounce like presenting them with a maze to traverse. This isn't because of laziness or a short attention span — potential clients might have already spent ten minutes perusing your content at this point — it's because frustration is a poor first impression, especially for clients who find technology intimidating.

So, whether you use an online scheduler or a virtual receptionist or prefer to get a phone call from every potential client, make this procedure easy, obvious, and ubiquitous. As clients scroll through your content, the opportunity to sign up for a session should always be plainly in view and as frustration-free as you can make it.

With some exceptions. While my sign-up procedure is fairly frictionless, I do require a name, email address, and phone number, as well as that click to acknowledge my policies. Clients will never see a same-day appointment, so everyone expecting instant gratification will bounce. You might require a street address or credit card number; both of these are fairly standard and will appear late in the process, so the likelihood of legitimate clients bouncing is low but non-zero. Just realize that this can be a good thing — it's nice to only see clients who are willing to comply with reasonable professional procedures. My goal here is to lose as few people as possible to confusion and frustration, and also to shoo away impulse clickers who aren't willing to make a minimal commitment.

Procuring plentiful, high-quality reviews. Seeing that "32 people recommend this business" or that you have "4.8 stars with 28 reviews" can be an instant confidence boost for potential clients considering that first appointment. It's even better when they scroll through those reviews and see people raving about how you found that perfect pressure and responded to their needs, or, that most excellent of compliments, that you have "magic hands." For a client who has had some frustration with the cookie-cutter massages they've been receiving at their local franchise, this can be like a sign from the heavens.

It can also be a source of frustration for a lot of massage therapists. You're getting return clients, you're getting glowing reviews in person, so why isn't anyone leaving a review online? I've got a hypothesis: it simply doesn't occur to them once they're back home, for the same reason we forget what we're looking for when we enter a new room. That specific phenomenon is called the "doorway effect," and it's a real and measurable reset of our working memory that occurs when we undergo a transition to a new setting. More generally, this is because of something called context-dependent memory: It's easiest to access memories in settings similar to those in which they were formed. This is why it's a good idea to study for the MBLEx in front of a computer screen in a depressing room that smells vaguely of old cardboard rather than on a bench at your favorite park. It maximizes context congruence, allowing for easier recall. That's a bit of a tangent, and I apologize.

The upshot is that we need to bridge the divide between when a client leaves our massage room, all aglow with the after-effects of a good session, and when they're next in front of their computer or phone. Those might as well be two completely different universes, so I like to give them a nudge in both settings. The first comes directly after the session: "Hey Susan, I'm trying to get some more reviews on my Google business page. Could I email you a link to that later?" The next comes via email, and this is my chance to influence the tone and content of the reviews I'd like to receive. "Hi Susan, it was great to see you today! Here's the link to my Google reviews, if you wouldn't mind leaving me one. I'm hoping to let new clients know how I'm different, and what sets my work apart. I appreciate you!"

This one-two punch bridges that divide between contexts, and it sets up the bigger commitment with an initial small commitment: "Do you mind if I send you an email?" This is called the foot-in-the-door phenomenon: Starting with a small request makes bigger requests more likely to be met positively. "Ian, isn't that a little manipulative?" Yes, and the more you know about social psychology, the more ways you'll learn to put your thumb on the scale to get the outcomes you want in business and health. Please use these powers for good rather than evil.

Invite your clients to plan ahead. As long as we're talking about social psychology, here's an important concept: Goods and services that are perceived to be in short supply are more likely to be valued highly by consumers. Goods and services that seem to be ubiquitous and unlimited are thought of as cheap and disposable. This is why it can be particularly damaging when massage therapists make themselves available to clients at all hours under all circumstances, always willing to make last-minute accommodations. The client's perception of your value decreases, and whether you're aware of it or not, your perception of your own value drops as well. This and other acts of accidental self-devaluation can be a cause of burnout, which we'll discuss in detail in chapter 9.

Instead, find ways to emphasize that you're a hot commodity, and that it might be wise to plan ahead rather than miss out on a preferred time slot. Start by building it into your policies: No same-day appointments, and canceling/rescheduling with fewer than 24 hours' notice can be subject to an appropriate fee. You can also build it into your public-facing availability: I like my appointments to be bunched together rather than having big gaps between them, and I prefer that the client only sees a few options each day, even if I'm not busy. Dig into your scheduling software's options to set your scheduling rules, and reach out to their customer service if you're not sure how to curate what your clients see.

Finally, encourage your clients to book in advance. That sounds something like this: "I'm starting to get booked out about a week in advance, so let me know if you ever want to reserve a regular time slot so that you don't get crowded out." Easy, no pressure, and it prompts the client to plan ahead rather than relying on happenstance. "But Ian, I only have a few appointments every week. What should I say about that?" Hey, that sounds like you're starting to get booked up to me! No, I'm not saying to lie, but do let your clients know that you've got a limited supply of openings, and that the only way to guarantee their preferred time is for them to grab it in advance, or even to set up a regular standing appointment. As you get more clients scheduling in advance, that will make the remaining slots even more scarce, prompting more clients to schedule in advance. A positive feedback loop!

"But Ian! If I don't give clients their preferred time or make other allowances for them, won't they leave me?" This is backwards thinking. The more allowances you make, the *less* loyalty you're likely to engender. Being constantly available requires nothing of the client, certainly not forethought or commitment. Asking them to meet you halfway by choosing from your current availability might lose you the occasional ideal client due to scheduling conflicts, but it will mostly get rid of the client tyrants who think their whims are paramount. You are allowed to have needs, and to create structure, and to set boundaries. That goes for your business life, and for your personal life. Let the tyrants bounce.

The invitation. This one is for massage therapists working in group settings, but the principle can be carried over to a solo practice. It's simply this: When a new client is about to leave and head to the front desk to check out, make sure they know that they're welcome back! This might sound obvious to some, but anxious folks like me get worried that we're "coming on too strong," so we engage in self-sabotaging behaviors like acting aloof and detached. This, as you might imagine, is a poor sales tactic. Worst of all, it's seen by some clients (anxious clients especially) as rejection, or even as an indictment of them as a person. "Oh, I guess I was a bad client. I'll just take whoever they give me next time and hope I don't get this therapist who hates me." If this sounds like exaggeration, then friend, I'm envious of your kind inner voice.

Instead of leaving them hanging, you can simply say, "I'd love to keep working with your low back pain, so please feel free to request me next time you make an appointment." This highlights your treatment plan, it's warm and welcoming, and it explicitly invites them to ask for you by name. This is enough to assuage the fears of the most anxious client, and it just takes a few seconds. When I was working at a massage franchise, this one little change was the catalyst that got me booked two weeks in advance!

Principles of effective promotions

While my focus has been on ads and an informative online presence, there are plenty of other useful strategies. Some of these require more extraversion than I can muster on a daily basis, but I frequently masquerade as an outgoing and confident guy when working at schools or in group settings. As you consider how you'd like to go about acquiring clients, there are some general principles to remember:

1. There are tons of potential clients out there who simply don't know that massage exists. "But Ian, of course they know massage exists. Everyone knows about massage!" Do they? They've seen people having their backs chopped in movies and on TV, but they've never even considered receiving one, let alone connected the idea with pain relief. Every time your promotions get served to one of these potential clients, you could be changing a life, and getting access to a referral network that no one else has tapped into.
2. You are not in competition with the massage franchises, and in fact, they will be feeding you clients. Because of the ways that franchises sabotage the therapeutic relationship, many clients will come away from that experience wanting something deeper and more customized. Every previously dissatisfied client is an opportunity to blow someone's mind.

3. Every promotional strategy is improved by repetition. Think about how many times you need to see a billboard before it sticks with you or prompts you to action. Doing chair massage at one race is unlikely to net you a single client, but doing chair massage at every race, every year? Soon people will start to recognize your face and your name, and when they just happen to come across your ad online, they'll feel like they already know you.
4. Every promotional strategy is improved by immediacy. Let me restate that as a negative: If a client can't act *now*, they're unlikely to act *at all*. So, no matter how you're promoting yourself, give clients the opportunity to give you money, to give you an email address, or to make a commitment. If you're introducing yourself to neighboring business owners, don't just pop in and say hi – give them the opportunity to sign up for a free sample massage while you're there.
5. Keep client quality in mind – you want your ideal clients, or clients who can refer your ideal clients. Casting too wide a net could garner you lots of clients quickly, but there will be a lot of poor fits who will have to be weeded out. By the same token, giving your services away for free or cheap can be effective, but that can easily attract bargain hunters and freebie foragers. Again, you'll be able to find your ideal clients from among these groups, but be careful about overloading yourself with clients who aren't specifically looking for you and your massage.
6. Seeking out a niche will always be more predictable than casting a wide net. Joining local runners' groups and becoming "that massage therapist that all the runners talk about" will net you a stream of high-quality clients, all looking for the work you've done with other group members. It's a low-stress way to go about things, and it can lead to powerful referral networks.
7. Networking with other professionals is a force multiplier. By this I mean: Having ten local massage therapists, acupuncturists, and physical therapists who all think highly of

you will lead to better outcomes for any and every promotional strategy you try. They'll always be in the background advocating on your behalf, just like you're talking them up and sending people their way.

8. Rapport trumps everything else. Rapport is the bond you form with clients and colleagues, and it's a combination of open communication and warm regard. If you have trouble opening up or untying your tongue, let time and repetition do their work on you, too. Even if you can't muster the courage to talk much during your first event, you'll be a rapport machine by the fifth event!

Other promotional strategies

With those principles in mind, here are some other methods to try:

Join networking groups. These usually involve paying to be part of a small group of professionals who each bring something different to the table; you might be grouped with a dentist, a chiropractor, a web developer, and a number of other business owners. To find these, just search "networking groups [my town]" on Google, and expect to find paid options like BNI and your local chamber of commerce, as well as free groups and events that can serve the same purpose.

How to make these work: Be an evangelist for massage, focus on how massage can be beneficial for your partners and their patients/clients/workers, and act as a useful networking resource. By that last one I mean: If they're going to be sending clients your way, consider being just as ardent in your support for them and their businesses. As always, let your best business practices and professional ethics guide what products you recommend and to whom you refer, but find ways to be an advocate for your new friends. Above all else, be consistent. Attend the meetings, be engaging, and make connections.

Make your own network. This might sound utterly mad to the introverts among us, but this option involves the following:

Sending messages or making phone calls to specialists and prominent healthcare professionals in your area and asking if you could meet them at their office and talk about their approach to pain. Reach out to physical therapists and chiropractors who specialize in the types of pain that fascinate you and ask to pick their brain and talk about their method. Do the same with fellow massage therapists who seem to have the same massage philosophy as you, which would sound something like this: "I'm just getting established here and I'm really impressed by what I've read about your therapeutic approach. Could I buy you a business lunch and pick your brain about massage?" Or, if you're an established specialist yourself (you get to decide when you're a specialist): "Hi X, I'm a fellow myofascial release practitioner and I just wanted to reach out, compare notes, and talk shop. Let me know if you'd be interested in a business lunch, or even a trade!"

Realize that the exact wording isn't important, and neither is whether you successfully have a meeting. Cast your net out, spend a moment to trumpet your own qualifications, and have a few lunches and meetings if people are willing. All this introduction and schmoozing has a purpose: You're getting your foot in the door with the local bigwigs and starting the process of establishing yourself as one of their peers. When they hear good things about you from a patient or client, they'll be much more likely to think, "oh yeah, that person is legit."

How to make this work: Seek connection and rapport among your colleagues, and once again, be a good member of this networking group. If you find a physical therapist who does really interesting work with hip pain, keep them on a short list of people to refer to when a client's pain is resisting full resolution. If you meet a personal trainer or yoga teacher who really seems to understand pain (and who won't push past someone's comfort level), the more clients you refer their way the better! Over time these reciprocal referrals and a developing regard for each other's competence will allow you to take your place among your city's pain specialists.

Drop off business cards and flyers. The oldest of the old school: Pounding the pavement and shaking hands. With this strategy you identify every business within a certain radius of your office, you stop by, ask to see the owner or a manager, and say, "I'm new in town and I was wondering if I could leave some information and coupons for you and your employees." Or, if you'd like to target that business's customers: "I was wondering if I could drop off some flyers and coupons for your customers." If you meet with the owner, you could offer to give them a free chair massage or shortened session as an introduction.

Once again, this isn't so much about having lots of individual successes, but rather seeding the area with your name and face. Some people will take your flyers, some owners will take a freebie massage, and everyone will know who you are.

This can be made even more effective by targeting certain businesses in a way that recognizes their needs. Leave flyers with dental practices and hair salons talking about hand and shoulder pain and how massage can help. Let that office complex know that you can help with wrist, neck, and low back pain. Police officers and nurses have aching feet, delivery drivers have low back pain in spades, and the workers at your local warehouse fulfillment center hurt everywhere. Type up a flyer addressing these concepts and the ways that you can help, attach a coupon for their first session, and include a link to your website for easy online scheduling.

Be everywhere, do everything. As far as word-of-mouth strategies go, this one is hard to beat. This means finding ways to be on committees, help plan events, have a massage chair set up at every event, and be part of every professional association. At these meetings and events you've always got your branded shirt on ("ask me about massage!" emblazoned on the back), you've got your fistful of business cards, and you're the most helpful person in the room.

To my fellow introverts: I must recognize, once again, that this sounds bonkers. But this strategy, and the networking strategies above, can all be self-executing like a computer virus, and self-propagating like a landslide. All you have to do is get started with networking and participating, and then *get out of your own way*. Whether you know it or not, you are surrounded by people who naturally follow the strategies above, and they all want to introduce you to their friends, and talk about the business community, and get you on committees. You will know these people because they will immediately start doing these things from the moment they meet you. Let the natural networkers carry you along in their tidal wave.

The trick here is to know when to say no, and to recognize your own limits. Working hard and being ubiquitous can make people rely on you heavily, so find a balance where you're consistently out in the community, but also keep an eye on your own capacity for physical and mental labor. If you're typically an introvert, you can look for work behind the scenes, like offering chair massage to an event's workers rather than to the public. Start with what seems possible, and let yourself expand from there if you find it fruitful and enjoyable. You can also...

Be everywhere online. This one's simple but potentially time-consuming, especially at first. Make a business page on Instagram or any other social media platform you feel comfortable with, then follow every small business and prominent person in your area. Then, start interacting! If that popular local food truck posts some beautiful brats and sauerkraut (with whole grain mustard), smash that like button and leave a comment about how amazing it looks. If the head of a local running club posts photos of their new puppy, leave a comment about how you would literally die for that perfect angel.

If you're a runner yourself, why not join that club's Facebook group and make the occasional post or reply? The same with your local mom group, or cosplay club, or Dungeons and Dragons forum. The point here isn't to insinuate your way into their good graces and then start posting about business, it's merely to be seen, and to be a part of your community. Every time you respond or like a post, people are getting to know your face and your name. "Hey, isn't that Ian, the massage guy?" You're darn right it is.

And make sure that people can interact back! Yes, post pictures of your massage office, selfies in your work outfit, and photos and videos of yourself in action. But also post pictures of food and sunsets and pets. Give people a chance to get to know you, and give them a reason to comment. While this might seem like a lot of effort just for a few internet likes, this can accomplish the same thing as being physically present in your community — as people pass your posts again and again, they'll become more likely to think, "you know, I do kind of feel like trying a massage." This can be a slow burn, but it's something that you can maintain when you're bored and waiting for a late client.

How to give away massage

This is something I've alluded to several times in this chapter, both negatively and positively. There's a reason for that: If you give away massage without a solid strategy, you'll just be spinning your wheels and devaluing the perception of your product. Giving a gift certificate to every charity in town is a good way to get a lot of thank you notes, but a poor way to drum up business. That's why you've got to hustle.

Let's talk about free chair massage, for example. This could be something that you get permission to do on a twice-monthly basis at your local gym, or in the nurses' break room at your local hospital. Maybe you do the same for your local teachers during teacher appreciation week. Here's how not to do it: Don't give a 15-30 minute massage that leaves the person drifting out of the room on a cloud of pure joy and relaxation. I know that might seem like a good sales strategy, but what you've just given away is the *whole experience*. It will feel like an amazing bargain, and the thought of then paying 90 dollars for something that they're used to getting for free will seem unthinkable. Instead, just offer enough of a freebie to leave them wanting more. Ten minutes is a good starting place.

Don't just "let your hands do the talking." Yes, massage feels great, and yes, I'm sure you've done a great job — they all say so afterwards! — but you need to let your mouth do some talking as well. As you're working, ask about any pain they might be in, and do a good job of customizing your pressure to their unique needs ("would you like more or less pressure than this?"). Take a moment to give your elevator pitch about how you treat pain, or your massage philosophy. When you're done, let them know that you'd be interested in working with that painful shoulder of theirs on the table, and that you think a longer session could really help. As always, just say what's true, and let that be your "sales pitch."

Finally, secure some form of commitment. This could just be an email address that you have them fill in prior to the massage. Useful, and it could lead to a future appointment! Even better is to say, "would you mind if I emailed you a coupon for your first appointment? I think you'd get a lot of benefit from a full session." Best of all is to ask, "would you like to go ahead and sign up for a session? I've got openings next week." Just realize that you can use your intuition here – if the client seems enthusiastic, go ahead and jump to asking them to sign up. If they seem lukewarm, then the emailed coupon is fine.

The same goes for shortened table sessions and other freebies that you might give away. Use that time to do a bit of talking and a lot of listening (rapport is the ultimate goal here), tell them whether you think they'd benefit from massage, and then follow your intuition as you seek commitment at the end. And even if the only thing you're consistent about is building rapport, you'll be infinitely more successful than someone who just silently gives away full sessions.

Becoming "that TMJ guy"

Before we go, I'd like to discuss a powerful strategy that can net you endless effortless business: Becoming "the person." The therapist. The guy. Becoming the go-to specialist on a certain aspect of massage or pathology, or even a certain type of athlete or business. My friends over at Massage Business Blueprint call this "niching," and they have a ton of podcast episodes on the topic for your listening pleasure.

This has accidentally happened to me a number of times over the course of my career. I'd do some good work with someone's jaw, and they'd tell a friend who'd come in for a session. Both would tell their dentist, and I'd start to see the occasional hygienist for their TMJ issues and arm pain. Here's the next step that I never take because I am incredibly lazy: I could have interfaced with that dentist, even asking one of the hygienists to introduce me, and I could probably have convinced them to start sending clients my way. This wouldn't be a business relationship, but rather an act of cementing myself in that dentist's mind as "our TMJ guy."

Do you do great work with the hips and sacrum, and one of your clients reports that they raved about you to their physical therapist? Ask for that PT's name and see if they'd enjoy a meeting of the minds. Maybe you'll find that you want to refer to them as well. Do this a few times, and you'll become "that massage therapist who does the good sciatica work" in your local PT community.

This doesn't have to be about referrals and happenstance; it can be a purposeful structuring of your business around a certain type of client or concept. Mention prenatal massage in the majority of your blog posts, feature it first and foremost on your website, and feature it in all your advertising. Before you know it, you'll be "that pregnancy massage therapist" that gets mentioned in every prenatal Facebook forum in your area (and you could participate on those forums as well). Clients will tell their friends, strangers will know your name, and obstetricians will start to hear more and more good things about you. This can easily become a self-accelerating process.

The tipping point

I've outlined a number of strategies above, some of which are rather high-effort, and some of which can be grown and tended in bits and pieces without much continuous commitment of time. I tend to prefer the strategies that I can do in dribs and drabs, but the ones that you choose will be up to you. No matter what, I recommend having an informative online presence, but the rest depends on what you feel drawn to, and what works with your personality and inclinations. If this reminds you of my philosophy of massage — there are lots of right ways to do things — then we're on the same page.

Keep that in mind as I impart the final business lesson: **Big things happen after the tipping point, and the tipping point eventually comes**. A *tipping point* in physics is when an object's center of gravity is far enough to one side that any further tilt (or the slightest push) will send it toppling over. Imagine a lamp teetering on the edge of a table. Well, something that I've found repeatedly in business is that things seem to happen slowly... until they happen all at once, in an incredible rush that can be rather dizzying. For two months you're plugging along, getting new clients via advertisements and word of mouth, and you're feeling like the tortoise racing the hare. Slow and steady, slow and steady. But imagine that there's a part of the fable where the tortoise teeters on a rock, flips over onto its back, and rockets down the raceway like a supercar.

That's how it tends to go in business. I'll be plugging away, slowly accruing clients, and then suddenly my schedule will be full. Or, I'll be plugging away, posting videos on YouTube, and suddenly I jump from a thousand subscribers per year to a thousand per week. I've noticed this phenomenon on all manner of social media, communities I've started, and even in personal endeavors.

So, what's happening? It's hard to say for sure because the process is rather opaque while it's underway, but here's what I imagine: All the work you've been putting in has been having secondary effects, and they reach a point where they become self-reinforcing. All the goodwill you've engendered in the community starts to potentiate your advertising. The clients you've worked on have told their friends, and those friends start to hear about you from other sources too. You pass a threshold where you're solidified as "that therapist that all the CrossFitters like." Or a combination of all of these, where each acts as a force multiplier for the others, and suddenly WHAM, you're flush with clients.

A side effect of this slow-then-sudden process is that it can be difficult to gauge the effectiveness of any given business strategy. Just like how a billboard doesn't really "work" until you've seen it a hundred times, most business strategies become more and more effective with time and consistent application. It can be easy to give up after a month of advertising if you've only gotten a single client, and it can be easy to give up on chair massage and interfacing with other professionals when they don't seem to bear any fruit. I'm just wasting money and spinning my wheels!

But remember the tipping point. You've got to keep nudging that lamp toward the edge of the table before anything loud and flashy happens. So, if that's true, how can you judge what's working? First, withhold judgment for a while. Let any given strategy play out for at least a month before you even think about changing it. Second, once some time has passed, look for little effects, even if there's no apparent acceleration. Did you get a new client from your flyers last month, and another one this month? Then keep at it, because you're inching toward something amazing.

Third, prune or tinker. Did you try a strategy for three months and the response is just completely dead? Consider trimming that one and refocusing on areas that have been more fruitful. Do you have an advertisement that seems sluggish compared to others that you've tried? Fiddle with it, read some articles and watch some videos on ad strategy, and see if some slightly different parameters make the interaction numbers go up. Remember, with online ads you can always post two or more and eventually get rid of the underperformers.

Finally, expect to pass the tipping point. Anticipate it, but don't grasp for it — just like all grasping behaviors, this can lead to self-sabotage. Instead, simply have faith that the little, incremental victories you've been having will eventually culminate in a disproportionate flood of success. Keep plugging along, keep making little alterations without prematurely pruning working strategies, and be playful as you do so. There are many roads to success in this industry, and each one reinforces the others, so you might as well have fun with it.

Again, does this all sound familiar? Because tipping points exist in therapy as well. A client might have dozens of small, temporary improvements over the course of months (which might even seem disappointing at the time), and then suddenly, their back stops bothering them at work. Another client might have ten headaches per week that seem resistant to treatment, until suddenly, something shifts and that number drops by half. Sleep might suddenly improve, or their mood will lift. Did you suddenly do something new that made this miracle happen? No, it was likely the culmination of all the good work you'd been doing for months.

Yes, discard strategies that are dead ends, and yes, keep tinkering and trying new things. But also have faith that the tipping point exists. If you're seeing those little victories, you can reasonably expect a big victory just around the bend.

Interlude: Business Resources

These have been my tried-and-true services for years now, but make sure to check the online supplement for links and for updated information: massagesloth.com/booksupplement

- **Canva**: This has been my ride or die graphic design service for years, and usually without paying a dime. Find the right size, add a nice background, add some text, then export as a picture file to post online, or a pdf to send to a printer. So easy it feels like cheating.
- **Vistaprint**: Cheap and easy business cards, magnets, and gift cards. Design on site, or upload your Canva creations. Make sure to search Google for "Vistaprint coupon" before you start, because there's always a deal going on.
- **Acuity**: My current favorite online booking service. Easy to navigate, lots of scheduling customizability options, and a friendly client experience that integrates well into Facebook and your website. Please keep in mind that a lot of online schedulers have similar functionality, and that all of them seem to offer a free trial so you can get a feel for them. Just remember that the client experience is most important, and that scheduling should be intuitive and simple.
- **Squarespace**: This is a site builder that also provides you with a web address (though that can be purchased elsewhere with some tech know-how). You pick a promising template, add some pictures and information, and you can even have a blog. They own Acuity and can integrate with it easily, or you can use whichever scheduler you like and embed it on a page. Other site builders like Wix are also good, and they all offer free trials. A site like this will cost a couple hundred bucks a year, and it's well worth it for ease of use and slick presentation.

- **Video editors**: A good video editor will be quick and snappy, letting you add graphics and text, and putting things in the right format for your social network of choice. Canva has started to offer this, or you can use CapCut on iPhone or Android (this is the video editor from the TikTok people, so it's very user friendly).
- **QuickBooks Self-Employed**: A monthly subscription that lets you classify your income and payments from multiple accounts as either business or personal. You can quickly upload pictures of receipts, and even track your business mileage using the app. At the end of the year, you can let your accountant view your data, check your work, and get your taxes done in record time.
- **Healthcare.gov**: If you're in the United States, you can likely get subsidized healthcare through the national marketplace at healthcare.gov. This is usually done during an enrollment period at the end of each year, but you can always sign up right after a qualifying life event, such as moving to a new state, or quitting your job at a massage franchise. Plans purchased through the marketplace are guaranteed to cover pre-existing conditions, as well as certain vital services like physicals, vaccinations, and well-woman visits.

Interlude: Business Q&A

How much should I charge? Enough to allow you to retire someday. And to take a week off every few months. And to enjoy your life. When you're pondering your prices and find yourself considering 50-dollar sessions, ask yourself: How much will this leave me at the end of the month? If it's not enough to feed your retirement fund and allow plenty of leisure, then you're selling yourself short, and borrowing from your future. If the only way to make the numbers work is to do 30 or more massages per week, then you might be setting yourself up for overuse injuries, or even burnout.

My advice when setting your pricing structure is to be bold. Look at what other massage therapists are charging in your area, discard the ones that are clearly trying to compete with massage franchises, and set your prices accordingly. If you're fresh out of school and still figuring out the ins and outs of running your own business, feel free to start out at a mid-range price, *as long as* this is still enough to pay into your retirement fund. Do this with your eyes on a gradual increase, and consider charting this out in advance. Rather than waiting for when you *feel* like an expert worthy of a higher price, throw that concept out the window and just commit to a plan for when you'll increase your prices. I recommend doing so once every year or two.

How do I change my rates or my hours? Ruthlessly! That's kind of a joke, but not really. The best way to increase your rates or change your availability is to announce it ahead of time, and to do so without apology or extensive explanation. Giving all sorts of reasons (e.g., comparing your rates to others, talking about your costs) or phrasing the change as an apology (e.g., "I hope this won't be too much of a burden," or "please let me know if this works for you") will make the changes seem random and capricious rather than well-reasoned and based on your professional judgment. Hedging and over-explaining can plant the idea in the mind of some clients that, hey, maybe this is negotiable.

Instead, keep these communications professional and brief: "It's a new year and there are changes ahead! My prices will be increasing as of [date], which you can see on my updated services list below." A lot of massage therapists will use this as an opportunity to sell a bunch of prepaid sessions all at once: "As a way of saying thank you to my current clients, any gift certificates that you buy before the price increase will be valid indefinitely, so feel free to buy as many as you'd like to lock in at the current price."

It's also a good idea to communicate these concepts to clients in person as the changes approach: "Did you see the announcement about the upcoming price changes? Your usual session will be ninety dollars instead of eighty, so keep that in mind." The same goes for schedule changes, especially ones that are likely to affect that client: "So Marie, as of March 31st I'll no longer be working Thursdays. I know those are usually your preference. Do you have any availability on Tuesdays or Fridays?" Keep in mind that, even if clients initially seem hard-pressed to find a time on your new schedule, most of them will adapt.

Before I move on, I'd like to acknowledge that making these changes can be scary, and it can be tempting to somehow cushion these blows, or to make lots of exceptions, or to make the changes as small as possible. Recognize that these thoughts come from a precarity mindset and dunk them into the sun. Yes, some clients might migrate away when you reduce your availability or increase your prices, but the ones who stay will be *more* loyal, and they'll be better evangelists on your behalf. Indeed, most clients will stick with you, so let that apocalyptic thinking float on by.

How do I enforce my cancellation policy? The best medicine is prevention, so make sure that it's stated clearly in places that your clients are sure to see it. I have my cancellation/no-show policy on my pricing and policy page, and on my scheduling page, and I make them check a box every time they make an appointment online to acknowledge their agreement to it. This can be stated fairly succinctly: "If you need to cancel or reschedule, please do so at least one full day prior to your appointment. Failure to do so will result in a charge equal to half the missed appointment cost."

From there, use your discretion. If a client is sick, that's a darn fine reason not to go to a massage (and we thank them for not bringing that into the office), so you can just say, "so sorry to hear that! No worries about the cancellation, just rest up and get well soon." If they don't have a reason, or if it's something like a scheduling conflict, you can choose whether to charge them for their first time. If you don't feel like charging for a first offense, that can sound like this: "I understand that some days just get out of hand. I'll waive the late cancellation fee, though I ask that you give me at least a day's notice in the future so that I have a chance to contact my waiting list."

But what if this is their second time, or if you'd just prefer to set a firm boundary and charge that first time? This can go two ways: You can charge the card you have on file specifically for this purpose (this can be set up in most online scheduling programs—just make sure to state this consequence explicitly in your policy), or you can send an invoice. Charging can sound like this: "Thank you for letting me know! You'll see a charge on your card for the cancellation fee. Have a good day, and I hope to see you soon!" Succinct, business-like. No need for it to feel chiding or like a punishment.

If you choose to go the invoice route, you can say, "You'll be receiving an invoice for the late cancellation fee in your email, please pay any time prior to your next appointment." And then... expect to never see that money, or that client ever again. The automatic charge with an on-file card will get you paid and might even maintain that relationship. The invoice that they can choose to pay or not? That can be a strategy. You see, I rarely enforce my late cancellation fee, because no-shows and late cancellations are unusual (most people are sufficiently chastened by the checkbox), and by the time I feel like enforcing it, I'd much rather be rid of the client than have their money. The "pay this invoice before you schedule" gambit is a good way to end a frustrating relationship.

However you choose to go about it, just realize that it's worthwhile to have a firm set of boundaries here, and that doing so is based on important values: "My time is worth money, and my mental health is worth more than money." You're not being a villain just because you expect timeliness and communication, and the clients who spend your time frivolously are not likely to be a good fit. Also realize that it's wise to expect some no-shows and late cancellations, and that they don't have to ruin your day. People are messy, life is messy, and it happens. Use the time to meditate and treat yourself to your favorite lunch, and keep moving forward.

How do I refer a client out? With love in your heart. I know that sounds weird, so let me unpack it: When we think of referring a client to another massage therapist, we tend to worry that the client will feel rejected, and so instead we trudge along, trying to fit this person's ideal. It can be wearying, especially when the client wants pressure that we're not comfortable providing, or they're dealing with issues that we're not well-versed in.

So, let your referral come from the same place as your massage: Acceptance, kindness, and non-judgment. You're recognizing your client's needs, and now it's time to help them get those needs met: "So Jim, I've been having some problems meeting your pressure needs, but I know a massage therapist who will be able to sink in and really work with your hip pain. If I gave you his card, would you be willing to give him a try?" Like most potentially difficult conversations, I keep this one brief and mostly clinical, but I also try to imbue it with the warmth I feel for this person. They deserve robust care that meets their needs.

What if your client still wants you as their therapist? Then this is a time to set boundaries, explicitly, out loud, with words. If you've been hedging around the fact that you don't feel comfortable with the massage they're asking for, now's the time to spill the beans. If you feel unequal to the task of working with their plantar fasciitis, now's the time to say so. As you go into these conversations, realize that your concept of what the client expects might be different from what they *actually* expect. They might not care all that much about ultra-deep work, or they might be fully satisfied with the progress on their plantar pain! Communicate early and often, and you won't be left trying to fulfill needs that don't actually exist, or that you're already knocking out of the park.

Okay, so how do I fire a client? If the last one was "how to send a client elsewhere without rejecting them," then this one is, "how do I exorcise a bad client like a poltergeist." This is for clients with whom you have irreconcilable differences, which might include constant lateness or last-minute cancellations; insistence on conversations that you find uncomfortable or even anxiety-provoking; constant boundary-crossing, such as sexual "jokes"; or even clients who you just dread seeing on your schedule. In any of these cases you might be able to salvage things by having a talk with that client. Let them know the problem as you see it (try "I notice that" and "I feel" statements), and then set boundaries. For the sexual "joker," that could sound like, "Harris, I've been noticing an increased frequency of sexual jokes and comments. Those leave me feeling devalued as a professional. I imagine that's not your intent, but it's how I feel. Would you be willing to leave those at the door while you're here?"

I know having these conversations can be scary at first, and that "scary" can be an understatement. It can help to allow these conversations to flow from your professional values: This needs to happen for the sake of the therapeutic relationship, so it's worth pushing past the anxiety. I'll practice in the mirror a few times, then I'll lay it out on the table. Be clinical and brief, don't worry if you stumble or say "um," and then simply wait. Don't try to anticipate how your client will respond, because that's a quick path to anxiety and self-fulfilling prophecies — imagine how different your delivery will be if you "just know" that they'll dismiss your concerns. Instead, let your client say whatever they'll say, and have faith that most clients will be willing to make reasonable changes when you express your needs.

Or, maybe it's past the time for talk, or you've *had* conversations that had no effect, or you're just ready to be done. In that case, I fully endorse using email or text to send the following: "Diane, the frequent rescheduling and late cancellations are negatively impacting my business, and I think it indicates an incompatibility between our schedules. I've canceled your upcoming sessions, and I ask that you seek future appointments elsewhere. Thank you for understanding." Or, in the case of Harris: "Harris, I've been feeling increasingly uncomfortable during recent sessions due to the content of jokes and comments that you've made. I've canceled your upcoming appointment and ask that you seek massage elsewhere. Thank you for understanding."

Yes, it comes across a little harshly, but you want the client to see a wall rather than a hurdle they can step over. Let your explanation be brief, focus on how you have been affected rather than on laying out accusations or evidence, and end with an unequivocal dismissal. There's nothing to argue with here, and many clients won't even feel the need to respond due to how final this seems.

Should I accept tips? If so, how do I get more tips? I see a lot of advice online saying to stop accepting tips — that such a policy will send a message of professionalism, and possibly act as a deterrent to creepers. While I agree with those ideas in principle, when I implemented that policy, I mostly just found it to be deeply frustrating to my clients. They *wanted* to tip me, and the fact that I wouldn't allow them to do so led to complaining and hilarious attempts to circumvent my prohibition. Clients were hiding tips where I'd find them later in the day, they were bringing me gift cards for coffee, and, I've got to say, I got a good haul of Christmas gifts that year.

When people experience something sublime, they want to recognize it, and just paying a standard fee feels equivalent to doing nothing. You could redirect this good will into ideal client behavior like reviews and referrals, but... I'd prefer to just allow them to tip! Engaging in loyalty-related behavior like tipping is likely to promote other such behavior, so preventing tipping could paradoxically *reduce* ideal client behavior by making the relationship seem more straightforwardly transactional. Social psychology is weird, which makes it worth pondering.

If you're not receiving much in the way of tips, it's usually a problem of opportunity rather than anything having to do with the quality of your massage. If you or your workplace rush the client through the exit process, or even make it automatic using a credits system, then there's simply little opportunity for the client to say, "wait, where's the part where I tip?" An easy fix for this is to just leave a tip plate in your room — this could be with a sign saying, "tips are never expected but always appreciated," or just an empty receptacle of some sort. This still leaves the problem that many people don't carry cash, at least not in useful denominations.

My solution for this, which works best when you're working for yourself, is to make tipping easy and available in each and every transaction. I'll say, "Alright Jim, that's 85 dollars for today. Credit? One second... okay, give me a fingertip signature and press the button in the upper right corner when you're done." I'll turn the iPad screen toward him, and there will be the signature line, along with four easy buttons that he can press to leave various tips. I don't mention them, but about 90% of clients know those buttons and what they do, and they tip.

If they hand me a wad of cash, I'll say, "can I get you some change?" I've never made change once in my life.

And if you do receive a tip, accept it kindly, and move on briskly. "Thank you so much! Now, would you like to go ahead and set up your next appointment?" People can feel a little embarrassed about tipping, and I find that a quick and gracious acceptance is enough thanks without seeming awkward.

How do I increase client retention? It starts with an invitation to return and the opportunity to book their next appointments on the spot. My retention numbers skyrocketed when I started asking the simple question, "would you like to go ahead and book your next appointment while you're here?" As always, no hedging, no implied apology, just a question. If they say yes, walk them through that process.

If they say something like, "I'll need to check my schedule," your response can be, "sounds good! You'll get an email later tonight with a link that you can use to schedule right online." In other words, whatever their response is, be brisk, be cheerful, and keep the process moving.

You'll occasionally have clients who kind of drop off the face of the earth, and it's easy to succumb to the idea that, "well, they must not have liked the massage." But about half the time, that client will mysteriously reappear eight months later, or you'll get a client referred by them who says, "man, Jane couldn't stop raving about you!" Huh? If they enjoyed the massage, why disappear? Why not set up regular sessions and soak up the benefits of massage?

Finances can be an issue, which is always something I'm sympathetic to, and one reason my approach doesn't involve any pressure or much upselling. But another issue is that *doorway effect* that we discussed earlier. Once clients leave the sanctum of our massage rooms and step back out into the busy and distracting outside world, they can effectively forget that we exist. A good massage can feel like an enjoyable dream — lovely and welcome, but able to evaporate from the mind like morning dew.

So, remind them! An email, *any* email on any topic, can be enough to get you a tiny flood of prodigal clients all booking at once. It can be news about a price increase or a schedule change, or just a notification that you've got some free spots in your schedule. It could also be a periodic reminder directed to that client, which can sound something like this: "Hi Jane, I hope you've been well! I've got some free spots this upcoming Wednesday and Thursday. If you'd like an appointment, you can click this link to schedule right online. I hope to see you soon!" A low-pressure nudge that is easily acted upon. If they don't respond to one or two of those, I just take them off my reminder list. No biggie — sometimes a client doesn't mesh with my style, and that just leaves more room for those who do!

You said something about upselling? I definitely upsell, mostly with a very specific goal: I want as many of my clients as possible getting ninety-minute massages. They're a better value than my hour-long sessions, they let me focus on every single trouble spot while also working with the whole body, and they're awesome. On my end, I do less laundry per massage hour, I get plenty of time to stretch my legs and flex my creative muscles, and it means less rushing to reset the room and reset my brain to prepare for a new client.

I do this in three steps: First, I stop trying to cram everything into the hour-long sessions, and I stop giving away free time to do so. Instead, I'll say something like, "James, we've got an hour-long session today and there's a lot of work I'd like to do with your neck and shoulders. Would you mind if we just worked from the hips up? I could still do a full-body session, but it would be fairly rushed." Say what's true, give them relevant information, and wait for their response. Most people will choose to forego the full-body treatment if it means getting a lot of focus on their areas of concern.

Second, plant the idea of longer sessions. "Let me know if you're ever interested in trying a ninety-minute massage. We'd have time to do more work with your hips and low back, and I'd be able to work with your whole body." This can be something you bring up as you wrap up, or even during the massage. You'll notice that this phrasing doesn't require a response. I just want the idea bouncing around in their head like a DVD player screensaver.

Third, as you set up their next appointment, say, "would you like that to be an hour session, or did you want to try ninety minutes? The longer session is thirty dollars more." Because you've laid the groundwork, it's likely that they've already made a decision here. Ask the question, and no matter what they answer, be brisk and cheerful as you set things up.

As for other upselling: Let your clinical judgment be your guiding light. Do you think they'd benefit from a reflexology add-on? Then say so, and then wait for their response. Do you have a product that you're fairly sure would improve their outcome? Let them know! As always, no pressure, just info rooted in experience and empathy.

What's the best way to do outcall/in-home massage? Planning to work directly in clients' homes? It's a great way to save on office costs, or to provide extra flexibility to clients in addition to your usual work. It can also be the only way that clients with mobility issues can receive massage, so offering outcall massage can be a matter of accommodating certain disabilities.

It's also somewhat likely to increase your creeper quantity, and to correlate with people pushing your boundaries in other ways. People see "outcall massage" and they think convenience and ease; these are concepts that are attractive to creeps, bargain hunters, and domineering types of all stripes. The solution here is to redouble your efforts to broadcast your boundaries, baking them into the booking process loudly and repeatedly.

Start by charging a hefty premium in addition to your normal fee — travel costs money, your time costs money, and the effort of setting up and breaking down can be fairly taxing. A single outcall can take twice as long as an in-office session for the same service, and should be priced accordingly. Then, consider charging in advance! This will seem standard to most people seeking in-home services, and it's something that any scheduling app will allow. Whether you use online booking or schedule by phone, I recommend having a policy against same-day booking, and sticking to your schedule. That might mean saying, "I don't have anything tomorrow, but I've got some availability next week." Is this likely to leave money on the table? Quite possibly, especially when dealing with tourists. It's also likely to nearly eliminate any potential creeper problem.

While these steps will filter out most ill-intentioned people, you might still choose to add an additional step: Make outcall appointments require extra confirmation. Most scheduling software will allow you to set services booked online as requests rather than hard appointments — make this clear during the booking process, and let the client know that they should leave a good phone number for a quick pre-booking interview. This can consist of, "what are you looking for in a massage?" and "do you have any pain that you'd like me to work with?" If there are any strange or probing responses, just say, "I won't be able to see you for this appointment. Thanks for understanding, and have a good day."

This might seem like an inordinate number of hoops to jump through, and indeed, it is likely to filter out some ideal clients as well. My recommendation is to set a high bar for unknown clients seeking in-home services, and to make the process much easier for your existing clients and their referrals. The newbies who make it through that first booking will be more likely to be there for actual massage, and you'll end up with a much less stressful life than if you had cast a wide net.

How do I employ other massage therapists? As peers. As fellow experts, rich in experience and knowledge that you don't have. As specialists who will be the best choice for certain clients, allowing each of them to find their perfect fit. When you hire another massage therapist, you're broadening the scope of your business, allowing you to serve not just a higher volume of clients, but also a greater variety of needs and communication styles. By recognizing your new massage therapist as a uniquely qualified expert and specialist rather than simply trying to slot them into a constrained role that you've created, you're treating them like a whole person and helping them realize their full potential.

Notice that this leaves little room for control and standardization. You might have a vision of a spa with a set menu of services which can be offered no matter who is on the schedule, but then you encounter an amazing massage therapist who does not offer 90-minute massages and who cannot tolerate essential oils. Should you discard the menu, or the person? You might want to hire three massage therapists who will each work five set days per week, but you find that you keep encountering candidates with availability that doesn't quite fit. Should you discard the schedule, or the people?

Consider this scenario: You offer $25 per hands-on hour, a full 25% more than the local franchise, but you still have nothing but trouble. Most of your candidates are former employees of that franchise, and they all seem a little burned out to begin with. You do your best to mentor them, but they still flake out on shifts, run late to appointments, and give poorly-reviewed massages. Your turnover rate is high, and so it feels like you're constantly spinning plates as you hire, train, and lose employees.

Now, consider this alternative: You offer $50 per hands-on hour, with pay increases for tenure and additional assistance for continuing education. This eats considerably into the $90 that you charge for a session, but after all, they're the ones doing the work. Even after business overhead, you still get paid well for the space you provide, the client base that you maintain, and the environment that you have created. In fact, you find that these massage therapists that you've attracted (some of whom are the same ones who would have burned out in the $25 scenario) help to co-create that environment. There's an openness and sharing of techniques that doesn't happen when people are fighting for a scarce resource. These therapists act as your evangelists, growing your mutual client base just by dint of their satisfaction and enthusiasm.

So, am I saying that money is magic and that paying more will solve all your employment problems? Yes. Yes, I am saying that. If you choose to be a massage employer, pay your therapists the lion's share of the value they create, and keep an amount based on the value that you create. This is a big part of how you forge your workplace culture: In a very literal sense, how much do you value your employees? From that foundation you can build extensions of that value — things like mutual support, reciprocal mentorship, and an open exchange of ideas. Think of the incredible value that each of these experts can offer when they find themselves in such a fertile environment.

How do I get rich as a massage therapist? Persist with the $25/hour scenario above, no matter how stressful and unsatisfying you and your employees find it. Put up with the last-minute schedule changes as employees call out or quit, and otherwise keep packing their schedules to the gills. Keep those résumés coming in, make presentations at your local massage schools to snatch up more new graduates, and lean heavily on the employees who put up with the abuse. Make sure to hold up those "rock stars" as a shining example of how an employee should act (everyone else won't hate this at all).

That, I'm afraid, is how you get rich in this industry. If you want to skip all the intermediary steps and get straight to the exploitation, there are multiple franchise companies who will happily let you buy in today and be up and running in a few months. You can make tens of thousands of dollars each month, just by the simple trick of rerouting most of the income from the people doing the work.

Or, you can charge for the work you do and the value you create, and allow that to suffice. You can do this as a solo therapist, setting your price at such a point that you're able to live comfortably and retire someday. You can partner with other massage therapists and open a larger facility with more versatility. You can rent out extra spaces in a larger clinic (though I ask that you base your price on the value you provide, not on the maximum that your renters can bear). You can teach, you can coach, you can make online content and create communities.

You can opt out of the paradigm that we've inherited, of maximum extraction with minimum investment. You can make sharing and generosity your bywords, having faith that others will respond in kind. You can secure a decent living and a respectable retirement, all while seeking quiet satisfaction.

Chapter 8: I Don't Know What to Say to Clients!

Imagine this scenario: You're just out of massage school, it's the first day of your first job in the field, and you've got three clients on your schedule. Client number one is set to arrive any minute now, and you're in your treatment room making sure everything is ready and perfect. Whether this is a distant memory or still in your future, this situation might have you sweating a bit. The massage part you can handle (all massage is good massage, after all), but what are you supposed to say? Okay, greet them, ask some questions... but what questions? What if they don't have any pain? What if they have very *specific* pain? What if you talk too much or mumble or say "um" a thousand times?

I've got good news and bad news. The bad news is that this isn't something you can just skip over and hope everything works out. Effective communication is necessary for robust consent, the prevention of medical errors, and establishing the rapport needed to allow your client to truly participate in the process. Massage is best applied with wide open lanes of communication, and it's incumbent on us as the professionals in the room to make sure crucial information gets relayed. Is the client actually comfortable on the table? Do they know that they can speak up about the pressure? Are they on board with your treatment plan?

The good news is that effective communication is mostly a matter of *time*. Yes, I do mean that it gets easier with practice and experience, but I also mean that *literal duration* is the most important factor for accomplishing your communication goals. Even if you don't have scripted phrases ready to go, even if you can't answer every question, even if you say "um" a lot or lose your train of thought – as long as you spend the time to have a conversation with your client rather than rushing through, you're going to do good, and you're going to do well.

The meet and greet

I don't want to overstate this, but the moment that you meet a new client will be seared into their memory forever, it will affect your entire relationship, and it could determine whether they refer twenty clients to you or just disappear completely. This is the make-or-break moment, the fulcrum upon which your destiny pivots!

Not really. None of that is actually true, and I wish we would stop telling people things like that. In fact, while first impressions are important, they're not nearly as important as lasting impressions. And here's the thing about lasting impressions: They're not based on what you say or how you say it, but on how the person *felt* as they left your office. It's about the time you spent and the care you demonstrated, and that hour-long session of feel-great massage that left them a little giddy. There are no make-or-break moments, and any verbal stumbles or missteps will be smoothed out by the flowing river of the total experience. In other words, communication is a distinctly *forgiving* process — if you find yourself stressing over how to say things in just the right way, I invite you to embrace imperfection and allow yourself to be a bit of a mess sometimes.

And so, as you go to greet a client, I don't want you to think of exactly what to say or how to say it, but to consider the feeling that you want to create in that moment: Welcome. Welcome to my massage practice. Welcome to my little world that I crafted just for you. Project warmth as you greet them, offer a handshake and a simple opening question, and help them realize that there's a process in place for this whole "first massage" thing, and that they can let go of their own nervousness about how to act or what to do in this unfamiliar setting.

For me, that sounds something like this: "Hi there, are you James? I'm Ian, nice to meet you. How's your day been so far? Great. I've got a short health questionnaire for you, feel free to take a seat right there. Can I grab you some water while you work? Alright, I'm going to go make sure everything's ready in my office and I'll be back in just a few minutes." Once I hear them click the pen closed or I see that they're done, I'll say, "All done? Alright, I'll take that clipboard from you, and we'll be right this way. Do you need to use the restroom before we start? We'll be right in here, just set your things down on that table and have a seat right there."

Brisk, brief, and straightforward. In my first ever meeting with a client, my goal is to project warmth and confidence, and to sweep them away with my established protocol. I don't want to leave them wondering if there's something they need to do or say – they're nervous too, and it's nice to know what's next!

Contrast this with a more scattered greeting that leaves a lot to the imagination. If you're a first-time client going to a new office based on a referral or an ad you saw somewhere, that can already be an intimidating proposition. What will you need to do? Who will this person be? If you step in and the massage therapist is talking to you over their shoulder as they haul laundry, leaving you standing in a waiting room without any clear next steps, you might be left feeling rather adrift. Should I grab that clipboard and get started on paperwork? Do I do something with that computer over there? Was I supposed to follow the massage therapist?

You can head off this crisis before it starts, and that can be a much more confidence-inspiring introduction to your space. Best of all, some of this work is already done via your website and social media – they know you, they know your office, and they might have even read your blog post on what their first massage will be like. From the moment this new client walks in the door, they realize that they can drop their worries and just look forward to a great massage.

A quick note on preconceptions

I talked about making your client feel welcome. Realize that this is only possible when it comes from a spirit of acceptance and non-judgment. A common phenomenon in medicine is that certain people receive less treatment than others and have a more difficult time having tests run or pain taken seriously. This is often true for people of color[9], for fat people[10], for LGBTQ people[11], and for poor people. When they walk into a doctor's office, they're much more likely to be treated as if the problem is all in their head, or a product of how they live. They're more likely to be suspected of malingering (i.e., "faking it") or drug seeking.

Now, imagine that you've been treated that way by doctors your entire life, starting from when you were young. Walking into a healthcare environment might seem like a time to man the battle stations and be on high alert for substandard care. Alternatively, you might feel resigned to poor care and feel detached from the entire process. To a new healthcare provider, you might come across as combative on the one hand, or sullen and withdrawn on the other.

So, imagine that you've got a client in your office who "gives you bad vibes." Imagine that they immediately come across as aggressive or domineering, or that they "just won't communicate," or that they "just seem to be another relaxation client." In other words: "Ugh, it's another problem client!" And maybe it was a feeling you had the moment they walked in the door.

That's when I want you to take a mental step back. To realize that you might be playing a well-worn role in a tale as old as time. Suddenly you're the healthcare provider acting distant or dismissive, being short and impatient, because "they're a problem client, and it's not like they'll book again." They act or look a certain way, so you act a certain way, and the vicious circle continues around and around.

I ask that you keep an eye out for this dynamic, and that when you meet this person who gives you "problem client" vibes, look internally and find your wellspring of grace and acceptance. Yes, this might end up being a poor fit. Yes, you should listen to your internal warning bells. But also make space in your heart, and in your practice, for those clients who might initially seem like a poor fit based on circumstantial evidence. You'll see that just by choosing not to play

---

9 https://www.forbes.com/sites/robertpearl/2015/03/05/healthcare-black-latino-poor/

10 https://www.ncbi.nlm.nih.gov/pmc/articles/PMC4381543/

11 https://www.ncbi.nlm.nih.gov/pmc/articles/PMC5478215/

the role of the dismissive practitioner, you'll frequently find a blossoming and fruitful therapeutic relationship on the other side. By choosing to cultivate non-judgment and be broadly welcoming, you'll find that some previously wounded clients are able to drop their walls and offer you grace as well.

The pre-massage intake

Now that you've projected confidence, you've kept things humming with your established first-time protocol, and you've had them sit in their assigned seat, there's something very important that I need you to do: I need you to tap the brakes, or even bring things to a screeching halt. A brisk pace was good for creating comfort and confidence during the initial meeting, but now that you've got them in your office, you've got a celebrity to interview. That's right, you've got the world's foremost expert on that client's body and their lived experience, right there in front of you. What an honor!

So, do what you'd do when interviewing an expert who you respect: Have a seat at their level or lower, rather than towering over them. Be ready with a notepad when there's crucial information, but make an effort to stay engaged with the conversation. When they have something to say, let them get it out without interruption. Once they're done, ask good follow-up questions.

All the above is important for a good intake, but my real reason for stressing the whole "interviewing a celebrity" thing is this: This is your first chance, and maybe your best opportunity, to really swing the power differential back in your client's favor. So far, they've had every reason to create an image of you as the expert in the room: Your knowledgeable online presence, your well-composed workplace, your brisk professionalism as they walked in the door. Now it's time to use that credibility you've created and extend that aura of power and expertise to your client.

This is also your first chance to open the channels of communication as wide as possible. Give your client implicit and explicit permission to speak up as often as they would like, with whatever they think might be important. When it comes to communication, you'll rarely go wrong by getting your client rambling.

So, what should the pre-massage intake consist of? Here are the high points:

1. A broad, open-ended question that lets them get their story started. "So Jane, what brings you in for a massage today?" If their answer is brief or doesn't yield any useful areas for follow-up, ask, "when you've had a really great massage in the past, what made it great?"
2. They might have a pain story to tell. As they do so, make sure to jot down all the different areas involved, then ask follow-ups to get more relevant details. "So, these headaches, how often do you get them, and where exactly do you feel them?" Make sure to follow up on areas mentioned on their written intake if they don't come up in the interview.
3. Broaden the scope of your questions to find possible leads. If they've got neck pain, ask about their shoulders. If they've got low back pain, ask about their hips. These likely pain associations are something that you'll become more fluent in over time, but if you're just starting out, simply ask about nearby structures.
4. Once you've gotten their story, it's time to give permission to speak up and to provide information.

Give permission to speak: This means letting the client know that you *want* to be informed if something needs to change, and that you want to be corrected if something feels off. For me, that sounds something like this: "So James, for this first session especially, I'd like us both to err on the side of too much communication. If I'm ever using too much pressure, just say, 'Ian, that's too much.' If you're ever clenching your teeth or holding your breath, that's too much pressure. If you're ever asking yourself, 'is this too much pressure?' — that's too much pressure. Okay? And the same goes for anything else that comes up or that feels important, never feel like you need to stay silent."

This is also when I would discuss any potentially invasive-feeling work I'd like to do: "Earlier in the intake you talked about pain here along your SI joint [here I gesture to the region on my own body]. I'd like to work right along that line and with all the rest of these hip muscles. Would that be alright? Okay great, just keep me posted, it should never feel like I'm in your personal space."

Provide information: Give them what they need to get on the table without worry. I don't want to leave anyone wondering where their clothes go, whether it's okay to be naked, whether to get under the blanket or sheet or both, etc. In other words, try to anticipate your client's concerns using your own experience as a client, and make this as smooth of a transition to the session as possible. Here's what my rap sounds like: "I'm going to step out of the room here in a second, and I'd like you to undress and place your clothes over there on that table. Naked is best because I would like to work directly with your hips, but if you choose to leave your underpants on, we'll work around them. You should feel well-covered at all times, and you should never feel a draft or anything like that. I'd like you to start face down on the table with your face in the face cradle, under the sheet and blanket. Sound good? Any questions, thoughts, concerns? Okay, I'm going to step out. Once again: Face down, under the sheet and blanket."

That might seem a little repetitive, and maybe a little convoluted, but it's what I've settled on over years of slight missteps and misunderstandings. I use the words "naked" and "underpants" specifically because they're explicit; when you say things like "undress to your level of comfort," that leaves a whole world of possible clothing configurations in the client's head, and it can make them feel compelled to leave more on than they otherwise would because they don't want to seem weird. So, rather than use polite language, I go ahead and ask them to be as naked as possible. I think that my verbiage above is encouraging without seeming pressuring, but feel free to make your own tweaks.

You'll notice how I mention starting face down twice, both in the middle of my rap and again at the end. That last parting reminder has brought my "successfully started how I wanted them to start" rate up to darn near 95%. As I discuss being under the sheet and blanket, I lift the top drapes to demonstrate. This, plus the repetition, has nearly eliminated the problem of people being on top of everything, cheeks bare to the elements.

Communicating during a session

The following might be a controversial opinion: Talking to your client during the massage is the best way to give better sessions, and to differentiate yourself in a crowded market. It can be the difference between giving a good massage and a great massage, and it's a skill worth developing.

"But Ian! Clients don't want me to talk their ear off the entire time!" This is absolutely true, but the only times I've ever heard clients complain about past therapists talking too much has been in the context of small talk, gossip, and sales. Having someone go on about work drama or politics for your entire session can be a unique brand of frustration, and being trapped on the table while someone delivers a sales pitch can make you want to wrap yourself in the sheet and flee the room like an Olympic sprinter. Relevant communication, the kind that enriches the overall experience and fits the feel of the massage, can seem like extra value. This doesn't need to be constant through the session (it might add up to 3-5 minutes of total talk), but just a small amount can amplify the effectiveness of your work.

This intra-session communication mostly falls into two categories: Session customization, and client education.

Customization: You've done some customization already, using the written intake and your pre-massage interview. You know the main areas of interest as well as areas to avoid, and you've discussed your initial game plan. That's an excellent start, but now's your chance to finetune your approach — and in doing so, find that perfect pressure, and home in on areas of profound importance.

Your client said that they like deep pressure, but that concept can vary so much from person to person as to render the term mostly meaningless. So, start with your idea of deep pressure, then ask the following: “So Jane, I’m sinking in here a little. Would you like more pressure than this, or less?”

You’ll notice that I didn’t ask, “how’s the pressure?” That’s because the answer to this question is always “fine,” even if the client can barely feel your touch. “Fine” is the polite answer, and it’s our job to bypass these social niceties and drill down to useful, actionable intelligence. As always, the burden of effective communication falls on us as the bodywork professional, which can mean pushing against our own impulse to be polite!

Instead, go with a forced-choice question: “Would you like more, or less?” The client can still choose to say that the current pressure is fine, but they’ll have to use more than a single word to do so, and they’ll have to think a bit before they answer. If they report that they’d like “a little less,” follow that with another forced-choice question: “Is this new pressure right, or would you like less than this?” Following this trail doggedly, especially at the beginning of your first massage together, can reveal the occasional client who prefers a tenth of your typical pressure, and who has never had another massage therapist actually interface with them at their level of comfort. Finding ways to dredge up the true answer rather than the socially acceptable answer is a skill worth honing, and one that will serve you well your entire career.

Encouraging fuller and more complex answers will also carry over to other areas. Once you’ve had a nice long pre-massage interview and established that you want full sentences on the massage table, you might find that your clients are more likely to provide actionable intel on their areas of complaint. To prompt this I might say something like, “Okay James, I’m in the general area that’s been giving you trouble lately. I’m currently looking for a really good spot, something that feels extra sensitive, or that really reminds you of your pain. Give me a heads up when I find that, alright?”

From there I’ll do some long, slow strokes exploring the area. If the client reports one of those important points, you can ask some follow-up questions: “What does that feel like to you? Is this too intense at all? Can you feel this anywhere other than right under my fingertips?” If that last question reveals referred pain, you can follow that trail by waiting for that referral to diminish (this is trigger point work at its most basic), by making contact in both places at once and inviting your client to take easy deep breaths, or by moving to the referral site once you're done with the original area. In all the above cases, you're integrating disparate areas of the body and telling them the story of how their pain works.

Education: Another use of communication during the session, which you can often integrate into the interactions we discussed above, is client education. This means finding key opportunities to make the body less confusing, or to give them context for techniques that might otherwise seem unrelated to their area of complaint. Here are some examples:

"This area that I'm sinking into right now is one of your rotator cuff muscles. Is there any sensitivity there? Do you feel that anywhere else, or just where my fingers are? Gotcha. These rotator cuff muscles actually wrap around the top of your humerus, your upper arm bone, so it makes sense that you're feeling this on the front of your shoulder. Go ahead and take some easy, deep breaths. Let me know if that sensation up front becomes less intense over time." As an aside, getting a clear referral pattern like that would lead me to a ten-minute detour of working with the rotator cuff thoroughly and with the arm in different positions. Moving on.

"Like I mentioned before the massage, I'd like to work with your hip region, which I think might be involved in that lower back pain you've been having. Will that be alright? Great. As I sink into this area, let me know if anything really stands out, either because it's extra intense, or if it reminds you of that pain you've been having. Right there? What are you feeling? Okay, take some easy, deep breaths. Right now I'm pressing near your SI joint, which is where a lot of your hip rotator muscles connect. It's pretty common for these to be tight in people who work at a desk for long hours, and that can be felt in the lower back. Once we're done, I'll give you some easy stretches you can do to keep these from staying tight all day."

The exact words in these examples aren't what's important, and neither is the smoothness of your delivery. Just taking the time to demystify the body and the way you're interacting with it can make the whole process feel like a collaboration rather than an operation. Instead of an expert applying inscrutable techniques for unknown reasons, the client is offered a window into your thought process, giving them a chance to provide more useful input, to refute a mistaken notion, or even to ask for a different approach. Best of all, they might stand up from their massage knowing that their rotator cuff is made up of *muscles*, and that those muscles can be influenced and stretched and desensitized. That's a much happier picture than when it just seemed like "some sort of cuff that I injured somehow."

Keep in mind that these questions and bits of narrative can be offered just as gently as any massage stroke, and that you can be just as intuitive and responsive as you would be with a technique. In other words, consider how to offer mid-session communication in a way that's friendly to the client's nervous system and congruent with the atmosphere that you've created in your office. If I haven't spoken for a while, I like to gently draw my client's attention with their name: "So Jane, I'm about to...", after which I speak slowly and confidently, using my "therapist voice." That's my soft, well-enunciated, slightly sing-song delivery that I find fits well with my massage setting, while also being comprehensible to someone who might be in a mild and pleasant stupor. If you're in a sports massage or medical massage setting, your therapist voice might sound more vigorous, or more crisply clinical.

As you approach the idea of including more mid-massage communication, you might find yourself feeling hesitant or embarrassed about speaking up. I ask that you treat this the same way that you'd treat any self-doubt about your skills or about trying new techniques: Acknowledge the fear, sit with it, let it fade, and then proceed with action based on intuition and experience instead. Self-doubt is normal, hesitancy is human, but you're committed to certain professional values and best practices, and effective communication is high on that list. Find your words, let them come out in mumbles and missteps if they need to, and know that by doing so, you'll be giving your client further permission to speak, and to be human.

How to make an exit

As you finish your massage, there are many right ways of capping off the experience, but only one wrong way. Let's start with the wrong way: You pat your client on the shoulder, say, "thank you!" and step out without another word. For one thing, this feels abrupt and incongruous with the gentle and flowing session you just delivered. For another, it sets up one of those miniature crises that we want to avoid: What do I do next? I should probably get dressed... but then, do I wait? Will they knock? If I leave the room, will I be able to find them? How do I pay?!

Yes, these questions will all be answered over the next few minutes, but not without some confusion and consternation that can seem like a dissonant final note to an otherwise excellent tune. Instead, make this last moment just as graceful and frictionless as the first. Start by bringing your massage to a close in a way that feels final. That can mean slow, rhythmic compressions of the draped back followed by fingertips sweeping down the body. It could be a long compression of both feet followed by traction of the legs. It could be a gentle cranial cradle where the hands slowly sneak out the sides. It could even involve singing bowls or Polarity contacts or slowly tapering body rocking. In any of the above cases, I recommend letting your final contact end slowly, gradually, and then allowing it to float away. It's a nice period at the end of the sentence.

From there, grab your client's attention, let them know what comes next, and then head out. You'll need to grab their attention to prevent them from drifting back into an altered state, or even to sleep. I like to say their name and ask how they're feeling, followed by some simple next steps: "Alright James, how are you feeling? Great. I'm going to step out of the room. Please take your time getting up from the table, there's no rush at all. As you sit up, if you feel at all lightheaded, please stay seated for at least a minute before you stand, okay? Once you're dressed and ready, just open that door over there and I'll have some water for you, and then we'll head to the lobby to finish up. Sound good? Great. Thank you!"

Kinda wordy, isn't it? Just realize that this is also a time for your client to come back to the real world and shake off the call of the warm, comfy table that's currently cradling them. My rate of needing to call out to slumbering clients through the studio door dropped by about 99% after I instituted my longer ending rap. It also answers questions that they might have about what to do next (seems obvious to us, but we're not returning from distant shores), it includes a needed precaution in case they're lightheaded, and it ends with an easy final step: I, the client, am the one who opens the door. You can shorten this in future sessions: "Alright, Jane, how're you feeling? Take your time getting up, no rush, and I'll meet you right outside the door whenever you're ready, okay?" Just keep it engaging enough, and thorough enough, that you can be sure they're fully rebooted.

Post-massage wrap-up

If mid-massage communication is where you differentiate yourself and generate a more powerful and customized session, the post-massage debriefing is where you make your money. It's where you set yourself and your client up for future growth and success. It's also where you take all the hard work you've done up to this point — all the work of creating an inviting and therapeutic space, the work of building rapport and opening the floodgates of communication, and the work of applying your contact in a mindful and methodical way — and bring it back full circle, wrapping your time together in a final layer of warmth that encapsulates and exemplifies the entire experience.

I know that sounds big and momentous, but think of how easy this last step can be. The connection has already been made thanks to your thorough interview and mid-massage communication, and that connection has been reinforced a thousand times over with every kind and confident massage stroke. If there's a sales pitch to be made or convincing to do, you've already done it, just by being an exceptional massage therapist! You accomplished these things without any high-pressure tactics, and without saying a single word about money, or discounts, or packages. If this person would like to be your long-term client, they already know it. If they're on board with your approach to treatment, they already know that too.

In other words, you're done convincing, and you're done selling. Now's the time to invite your client to do whatever it is that they've already decided to do. Invite simply, invite confidently, give them the honest assessment of your clinical judgment, and do so without self-sabotage.

More on that in a second. First, let's welcome our client back to the world of verticality and full-strength indoor lighting: "Hey Jane, welcome back. How are you feeling? Awesome!" As your client emerges, be aware that this can be just as intimidating for them as when they first stepped into your lobby. They've just had this incredible conversation with a stranger, mostly silently, and now they're encountering you again. It's like seeing a teacher at the grocery store — do we still have the same relationship in this other place? Are they happy to see me? It's a boundary between worlds, and it can be nice to instantly know that you're still welcome, and that the warmth is still there.

Second, follow up on their areas of complaint. "How's your neck feeling?" I like a nice open-ended question here rather than anything too specific. I want their trip report, and I don't want to lead the witness. Whatever they volunteer, they volunteer. From there you can offer self-care advice, as well as lay out your vision for their future treatment: "So, I think we found a useful direction for working with your neck pain today. In future sessions I'd like to keep exploring that levator scapulae muscle we talked about, and do more to open up your chest. If we could reduce the frequency of these cricks, that would be awesome."

Third, take your payment (if this is done by your front desk, skip to the next step). Do this with the same crisp professionalism that you showed when they walked in the door: "Alright, that will be 90 dollars today." If they offer cash, ask, "can I get you change?" If they use a card, I like a system that gives them big buttons they can press to offer a tip, but otherwise I don't mention the topic: "Go ahead and give me a fingertip signature on the line there, then hit the blue button in the upper right when you're done." For anyone who leaves a tip, I offer a brisk, "thanks so much for that, I really appreciate it," then move right along. I talked more about tips in the business Q&A before this chapter, but my general strategy is this: Give people the opportunity to tip, be gracious if they do, then move past it. People want to tip, but they can feel somewhat awkward about it. By making it just a quick footnote to the payment process, I'm able to relieve the awkwardness while still affirming that, yes, I am happy to receive recognition for my artistry, thank you.

Finally, invite your client to come back, and reassure them that you'd be happy to have them. This is the step where you can choose to empower your client to express the choice they've already made, or sabotage yourself by leaving them feeling unsure of whether you're fully on board. "But Ian, of course I'm on board! I love when clients come back!" Then why do we sometimes end up sounding hesitant, or even dismissive?

Sloth-style sales

When I think of the sales style that I've ended up with after fifteen years, it can be summed up with this general ethos: Be inviting, and don't get in your client's way.

Consider the post-massage client. They just enjoyed a great experience, maybe something deeply moving or just plain enjoyable. Their body is moving smoothly, their brain feels like it's been dipped in molten chocolate, and they've already figured out that this could be a good addition to their life. Their new favorite person has caught them like a lobbed ball and gently ushered them through a little conversation and a frictionless payment, and then... nothing. The therapist closes up, or says goodbye, or seems distant. I guess it's time to leave? Maybe I was a bad client.

The interval after a first massage, especially, is a time of vulnerability. It's a state that franchises like to prey upon by plying them with discounts and if-you-sign-up-now offers and well-practiced sales pitches that end in a contract that they barely remember signing. We don't want to be like that, and we don't want to seem "salesy." The thought of pressuring someone is so alien that, well, we'd rather go in the other direction entirely: "Thanks so much, you can make your next appointment online, if you want to. Have a nice day!"

Consider that client, happy but vulnerable, suddenly getting shunted out of the office. They thought they'd made a connection, but maybe they were wrong. Maybe their presence was an imposition. Maybe their body was too much work, or too weird, or had too much hair.

This might seem like I'm making a mountain out of a molehill. We've done all the convincing we need to do with our session, right? Well, there's a final question left in the client's mind, one that we can't leave unanswered: "Am I wanted?" They've just bared their body, an act of vulnerability that isn't easy in any context. That act was met with affirmation and kindness, but it can still leave people feeling off kilter once they're out of that sanctuary, that alternate reality.

So, instead of letting insecurity and self-doubt determine my sales style, I rely on a much more solid foundation: Say what's true, ask the client what they'd like to do, and then allow them to do the rest.

Here's what's true: Your client could benefit from massage. It would be a positive addition to their wellness regimen, and they'd be well-served by making room for it in their lives. If you have relevant insight from your clinical experience or your reading of the research, you can use that to make a more specific recommendation for session frequency, tying it to certain expectations you have for their symptom trajectory. I then ask them what they'd like to do, and then I wait for their answer. For me, that sounds like this:

"So James, when I'm dealing with frequent headaches like yours, I like to start with weekly massages and then space them out more as your symptoms become less intense. In my clinical experience, that usually takes about four weekly sessions to get that ball rolling. Is that something you'd be interested in trying?"

And then, I wait, without attachment or expectation. Remember, your client has long since made their decision, and you've done all you can to shift the power differential back in their favor. By asking plainly and explaining your reasoning, you're doing right by your business ethics, and you're refraining from poisoning the well with needless prevaricating or hedging.

Compare this with asking, "do you think you'd like to come back? Only if you want to! We could try once a month and see what happens." This sounds like you're unsure of your own profession, of yourself, and of your ability to get results.

"But Ian, I really am unsure whether massage will be effective for some clients!" Then, once again, say what's true, and be as tentative as the situation warrants: "I'd like to start you off with more frequent sessions to see if we can make a dent in your back pain, preferably once every week or two weeks. If my approach can help with your symptoms, we'll probably know after the third or fourth session. After that we can put our heads together and decide how to proceed. Is that something you'd be interested in setting up?"

If your client is just there to relax, or to de-stress, or for the sheer joy of massage, you can simply say, "I'd love to see you back as often as you want to be here. Would you like to go ahead and set up your next session?"

From there, the rest handles itself. They're either on board with your treatment plan, or they're not. They might have questions or want to know whether a lower frequency would work (my answer: "Any massage is better than no massage, and we can keep touching base about self-care when I see you."). They might give a polite deferral like, "I'll need to get home and look at my schedule." Not a problem! Here I respond with, "sounds good! You'll get a follow-up email later today, and it will have a link that you can use to make your next appointment at your convenience."

By succinctly stating your recommendation and asking them how they'd like to proceed, you can end this session how it began: With warmth, with quiet professionalism, and without judgment. Whether they sign up for their next session or demur, they'll leave your office feeling well cared for from beginning to end, and know that they're welcome to return. They'll feel that they were heard and responded to, and treated as a partner in their own healthcare. Best of all, they'll feel *good*, and the experience in its totality will supersede anything you said, or forgot to say, or stumbled over. It can be as easy as that.

Communication best practices

Before we move on to common client questions, let's talk about best practices for communication. Some of these were implied in the examples in this chapter, but I think it could be useful to state them explicitly. These aren't set in stone, and you can always adapt based on each unique therapeutic relationship that you forge.

1. **Clarity and connection are more important than precision**. In other words, it's more important that you be *understood* than that you correct every misperception, or that you use precise anatomical terminology. If a client uses the word "knot" and doesn't seem to have any self-stigma about it, I'll follow their lead. I can expand their awareness of that pain and tightness over time, but at first, it's more important that we speak the same language.
2. **Be judicious with jargon**. This follows from the rule above: Only use complicated terminology when it helps the client, and do so with plenty of context. It can be hugely illuminating to learn that there's a muscle called "levator scapulae," and that it connects the neck to the shoulder blade. It helps the client realize that there is a specific culprit for their cricks, and that it's not just some general "neck problem." When you introduce such terms, surround them in a cushion of easily understood explanation, and don't overwhelm the listener.
3. **Use the power of silent attention**. As you go through your first ever interview with a client, give them the full spotlight of your attention. Meet their eyes, give them a nod when they seek to be understood, and otherwise... wait. Don't pounce with follow-up questions or comments the second their story seems to be slowing. Instead, use your intuition as a guide and give them extra time when they may need it. Let there be a

momentary silence if they seem to be searching for their next thought, or if they're on a roll. Let them tell their story.

4. **Don't lead the witness**. As you ask questions about pain, do so without eagerness or attachment to the answer. Clients want to be cooperative and to please healthcare providers and scientists (a phenomenon so powerful that it can ruin otherwise good experiments), so try not to give clients the idea that affirmative responses are the "correct" answer. When they report pain, nod and make a note, and ask good follow-up questions without undue enthusiasm. When they say, "no headaches lately," nod and move along briskly, without acting surprised or otherwise dubious.
5. **Mirror emotion and intensity**. While the foundation of your interactions with clients can be mild clinical detachment and nonjudgment, as above, there are times to let your empathy shine through. If a client describes how their pain keeps them up at night, or keeps them from their favorite activities, you can choose to dip a toe in the river of their experience and feel that pain and frustration with them. This might be expressed with something as small as a furrowed brow and an empathetic nod, and this can let your client know that you recognize the gravity of their situation. You might also choose to say, "that sounds really difficult," or, "I'm sure it was hard to give up your music," or just, "I'm so sorry." You don't have to dig, and you don't need to act as a counselor, but there's no need to shy away from connection and shared pain.
6. **Always engage in your best practices, no matter the client**. When I go see a new massage therapist, I always appreciate being treated with thoroughness and care, even when I "should know the drill." Don't skip over important bits just because your client has gotten plenty of massage before, and don't inundate nurses and dentists with anatomical jargon. This is a new context, they're not at work, and it can be nice to have a soft landing in this new space. Thorough communication, delivered kindly, will always be a good way

to welcome a client, whether they're a fellow massage therapist, a doctor, or your own dear mom.

And, of course, feel free to make changes as you feel appropriate. I'm always thorough in my initial session, but I allow the intake to be shorter and snappier in subsequent sessions. If there's a long conversation, fine; if not, that's fine too. Let clients lead the way, and be willing to wrap up an interview if the client doesn't have a story they feel like telling that day. All we can do is create the right circumstances and do our due diligence. Connection and open communication can be facilitated, but they can't be forced.

The only time I'll press for more communication from a taciturn client is to prevent medical errors. That means that if a client isn't forthcoming about the details of their recent surgery, I'll persist until I have the information I need to make a sound clinical decision. If a client is responding "hm" to my questions about pressure, I'll stop the massage if necessary in order to explain why I'm asking and attempt to get useful answers. It's better to come across as rude than to be left saying, "but she never said the massage was painful! She should have spoken up!" As the professional in the room, the burden of effective communication and informed action always falls on us.

Interlude: Common Client Questions

Why am I in pain? I haven't changed anything. Sometimes tightness and sensitivity can creep up in the background, and you only become aware of it when it crosses a tipping point, and then you're *very* aware of it. The good news is that we probably just need to get it out of this crisis state for the pain to subside, but we'll also need to work with the months or years of tightness that may have predisposed you to pain in the first place. It would be nice to prevent this from cropping up again!

Why does my right side hurt and not my left side? It can have to do with how often you use each side, which side you carry your purse on, things like that. Sometimes it almost seems random. I often find that even though only one side is speaking up, people seem to be pretty symmetrical. That's why we'll explore the painless side as well, just to make sure problems aren't starting to develop there.

Is there anything you can do to help with post-workout soreness? Yep, massage can be pretty effective for reducing delayed onset muscle soreness (DOMS)[12]. It won't prevent it completely, but it might make the experience less intense.

Can massage help with my athletic performance? It can be a good add-on. Your training sessions are powerful stimuli for your muscles and nervous system, but too much of one type of stimulus can eventually lead to injury or sensitivity. Think of massage as cross-training: A different kind of stimulus that talks to the nervous system in a different way, helping it keep things in perspective and not overreact to your training regimen. It might not help your performance directly, but it can make you more comfortable in your body as you train[13].

Should I try to stretch this out? Sometimes stretching can help with injury recovery, especially once you're out of the spasm

---

[12] https://www.ncbi.nlm.nih.gov/pmc/articles/PMC5932411/
[13] https://bmjopensem.bmj.com/content/6/1/e000614

stage and into the stiffness stage. Just be gentle and gradual, and think of it as a conversation with your nervous system. You're not trying to stretch taffy, but rather sending the signal that this muscle is capable of safely extending. But if your back "goes out" and you're in a world of hurt, don't try to stretch that out. That's the time for rest.

Should I use heat or ice? Both are good! Neither of them has a huge effect on injury recovery, but each can have a small analgesic effect. I avoid heat for straight up trauma like a twisted ankle, but for muscle spasms and tweaks, it's my preferred way to mellow out the area. I like ice for joint pain, but if you prefer heat, go with what works for you. You can also try contrast therapy, which is where you apply heat and ice in an alternating fashion. If I tweak my back, I'll lie on a heating pad for 30 minutes, switch to an ice pack for 10, and then go back and forth a couple times until the pain and stiffness have reduced.

What's a trigger point? It's a little area in your muscle that tends to be extra sensitive, and sometimes it can refer pain elsewhere. It's not something we can get rid of, but we might be able to reduce that sensitivity and referral.

I keep waking up with a stiff neck. Do I need a new pillow? A new pillow might help, but when I hear about frequent neck stiffness, I'm thinking about how that person spends their day rather than their night. In other words, is there anything you do during your day-to-day life that might be predisposing you to neck tightness or irritation?

(From here, I'll talk with the client about their desk ergonomics, or their body mechanics while cutting hair/cleaning teeth/fixing cars, etc. A little mindfulness about neck tilts and forward head posture can be a relief for their levator scapulae. From there I recommend some gentle stretches for the pecs and neck; the more protracted their head and shoulders are, the more work levator is having to do while staying elongated.)

Why is my joint crunchy? That's something called crepitus, and it's fairly common in people with no other symptoms. If it's causing you worry, or if there are other symptoms like pain or dysfunction, then bring it up with your doctor.

My doctor says I have a slipped disc/arthritis. Can massage help? Probably, yes. Even if your pain has a clear structural component, there will always be some involvement of the local muscles and nerves. I won't be changing the structure, but if we can calm that high tension environment in your muscles and convince your nervous system to lower its sensitivity, we can reduce your pain. Lots of people with some degree of disc pathology or arthritis live without any symptoms at all, so hopefully that's something that we can work toward.

(The same goes for scoliosis, labrum tears, acromioclavicular joint dysfunction, and all manner of degenerative joint disorders. There will always be a nervous system element to any pain, conservative/non-invasive management is often as effective as surgery[14], and there will almost always be a wide spectrum of pain and dysfunction among those with similar structural differences. This can mean that people with similar degrees of joint space narrowing can range from fully disabled to completely asymptomatic. This leads me to believe that there are functional elements that we can influence, even in the presence of structure that we can't change.)

---

[14] https://pubmed.ncbi.nlm.nih.gov/28253054/

Chapter 9: I'm So... Burned... Out

This chapter is for all my colleagues who have lost that spark, that special feeling they had in massage school where it seemed like massage was magic and anything was possible. Even worse, massage has started to feel like a slog, like pushing a boulder uphill only to watch it roll back down, day after day, week after week. Are we even accomplishing anything? Are we just a temporary fix, a feel-good distraction? What's the point?

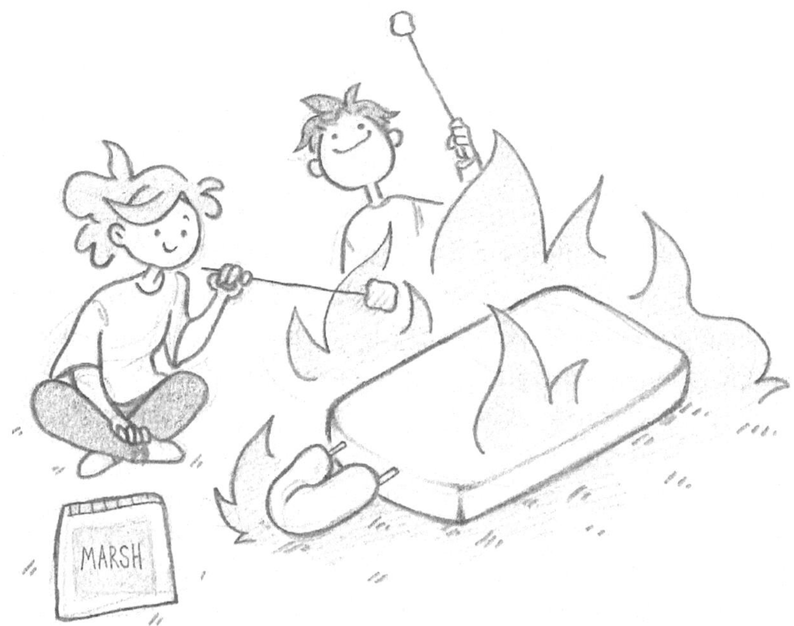

My friend, you might be experiencing something that industrial/organizational psychologists call *burnout*. It's experienced in every field, in every vocation and calling, and it doesn't matter whether you're doing research in a lab or art in a studio, it can make you question whether you're actually doing something worthwhile or just spinning your wheels. It can make you feel like your work has no meaning, and it can rob you of the joy that used to feel so natural, the intrinsic motivation that felt like an immutable feature of your vocation.

Well, massage *is* magic, and anything *is* possible, and I want you to be able to reconnect with that feeling. That half-mad, kid-in-a-candy-store feeling that you had in massage school where there were a hundred modalities to choose from, and the secrets of the tactile universe swirled around your head. You were right to have that feeling, and you can get it back!

All you've got to do is shed some layers. Without realizing it you've acquired some baggage that's weighing you down, and you've piled all sorts of thwarted expectations and self-imposed rules and negative experiences on top of your old joy. It's still there, a vast resource of playfulness and curiosity just waiting to empower your work and rocket you to new heights, but first we've got to peel away all the junk that's plugging your well. Let's get to digging.

The perverse incentives of capital

When you research burnout, you'll see all sorts of potential causes and well-meaning solutions, most of which fail to mention the most obvious source. People will tell you to reconnect with your work, or change your room layout, or take a class. They'll say that your work-life balance is off, and maybe you should take a vacation!

These are all good ideas (and indeed, we'll talk about some of them later), but from my 15 years of connecting with therapists and working in the field, I've got a major suspect in mind, and it's not simple stagnation. It's an oppressive, exploitative work environment that's strip-mining your enthusiasm in the interest of making as much money as possible with minimal investment, all to repeat the process with someone new once you burn out like a meteor.

I'm talking about crappy bosses. Franchise owners who rush you through a ten-minute orientation before piling your schedule with six massages in a single day. Chiropractors who think that you can somehow work eight hours straight without your head or your hands exploding. Work environments where you're somehow expected to conduct meaningful intakes and keep thorough SOAP notes while only having ten minutes between clients.

And it can all seem fine at first, even bracing and empowering. This is a challenge, and it turns out your body is up to the task! You take on those weeks with thirty plus hands-on hours and find that you're able to get into a groove: You slide into work, see your full-to-bursting schedule, and knock it out like a champ. Then you head home, grunt a greeting to your family, and collapse into a recliner with just enough energy left to pull the lever. Eventually, you start needing to ice your forearms when you get home so that they hurt less the next day. Rinse, repeat, ad infinitum until the end of the universe.

Over time, you start to feel alienated from massage and everything it used to represent. The work itself can start to feel pointless and even oppressive, and it can be easy to get into the habit of resenting your regular clients, but not half as much as you resent newbies (damn them for throwing off your schedule!). Each session is a box to check, and once you check three more boxes you get to go home. That day's slog represents about a hundred and thirty dollars, maybe a hundred and fifty with good tips (damn those bad tippers!).

If any of this feels familiar to you, I just want you to know that I've been there too, and it's not your fault. You've been put in an untenable position, one that is completely antithetical to the idea of a therapeutic relationship, or rapport, or the creation of a nonjudgmental sanctuary. By treating you like a cog in a money-making machine instead of a valued expert in your healthcare field, your workplace has robbed you of professional dignity. By asking you to treat new clients like prizes to be won, and involving you in a coercive scheme to procure year-long commitments using the very power differential that we should be working to minimize, you're being manipulated as well.

Drama, competition, and winning

That's not to say that overwork is the only villain in this tale. Underwork can be just as draining, especially in an environment where there are winners and losers. When I first started at a massage franchise, I spent a lot of time sitting in the back room, either twiddling my thumbs while waiting for my second and final appointment of the day, or hoping that I'd be assigned a walk-in. While I was back there, I was surrounded by my fellow laggards, all of whom felt somewhat disaffected by the indignity of it all. Why do John and Joan get all the walk-ins when they already have so many clients? Why does the front desk hate us? What's management's problem with me? This was an environment ripe for gossip and backbiting, and it was the toxic stew that every new hire was at least briefly dipped into during slow shifts. It engendered a cynicism that could easily follow you into the massage room, or even stick with you for the rest of your career.

The only escape from this rogues' gallery was to be one of the winners: Ingratiate yourself to the front desk, start pumping up your member conversion and upselling numbers, and become one of those lucky few who was swamped with clients. Once you "won," your prize was more work and longer hours, and more walk-ins crammed into the space where your lunch break was supposed to be. This is because the front desk and management are operating under perverse incentives as well: They're not there to look out for each employee or ensure equal treatment, they're tasked with taking a 75% sign-up rate and turning it into 76%. This leaves very little room for individual consideration, or the simple kindness of treating a working body as anything other than invincible. I saw many good massage therapists worn down and injured by this paradigm, some of whom are lost to the profession forever. They burned out.

And for what? At my peak at the massage franchise, when I was slammed and keeping my numbers at the top of the performance list and successfully upselling truly dreadful aromatherapy treatments, I was making about 1400 dollars per paycheck. That's about 33,000 dollars per year before taxes, painstakingly earned 20-30 dollars at a time, session after session, week after week. My body ached, I had injured my right thumb in a spectacular fashion, and, crushingly, heartachingly, I was at the top of my game. This was the mountaintop, and there was no way to move up from there other than to abandon my client base entirely and start over. They had pitted me against my fellow workers, they convinced me to give my all in service of a membership program that I found unethical, and they'd even had me sign a non-compete clause that ostensibly meant I couldn't work in my own town after quitting. I had never felt more burned out, and it made me wonder: Was massage a mistake? Was it ever worthwhile? Is that all there is?

Habits of highly horrible bosses

Just so that we're all on the same page, here are the typical tactics of a terrible boss:

1. **Always on call**. This is a favorite behavior of abusive bosses: Always expecting you to be able to hop to, all without paying you for the massive disruptive effect this has on your life. This can take the form of unpaid "on-call" days, or just a general understanding that you might be expected to fill in or "help out" on any given day. You want to be a team player, right?
2. **"Sure, we can fit you in."** This goes hand-in-hand with disrespecting your time and the sanctity of your body: Finding that, at the end of a long day with five hours of hands-on time, you've suddenly got a sixth client, and they're in the waiting room already! It's a rather crushing feeling for someone who was already running on empty.
3. **Side work doesn't count**. All the cleaning and paperwork is uncompensated and unrecognized. It needs to be done, it's *basically* part of the hands-on work, so let's pretend that it's not taxing and time-consuming!
4. **"Why should I thank her? I pay her!"** That's an exact quote from the worst boss I ever had. My answer to this question: We are paid because we work. We deserve recognition because we're experts. We deserve kindness because we're human.
5. **Keeping you hungry.** This is the most insidious habit of a bad boss, and it's not necessarily about money. It's the *feeling* that your employment situation is precarious, and that the only way to feel secure is to push harder. Push for those extra upsells, be willing to change your schedule on a whim, pump

> those numbers up. You see how poorly the worst performers are treated, and you're regularly reminded that you're on the bubble.

These are the big overt behaviors, but realize that a draining and degrading work culture consists of a thousand small indignities as well, all of which accumulate over time and can hang off of you like sandbags. Here I'm talking about the short snappish commands that are better suited to interacting with a voice-activated speaker. The tag-teaming with multiple managers who all feel the need to point out a shortcoming (think "TPS reports"). The passive-aggressive stomping around that leaves everyone on edge and hiding in the back.

As you consider these behaviors, I want you to zoom out and look at the bigger picture. No one sets out to create such a precarious and chaotic environment, and few people wish to be feared and hated. This deeply toxic workplace developed over time — these bosses probably started out trying to be gregarious and kind, but found that they needed to keep a tighter leash on their employees. They just keep not showing up to work, or quitting after two weeks! And these front desk employees are so lazy, I need to start cracking the whip! The phrase "it's like herding cats" probably passed their lips more than once, especially while trading tips with their fellow business owners. Massage therapists! Who can work with these flakes?

They turned themselves into petty tyrants because they felt like they had to. How else can you get consistent, high-quality work while keeping 75% of the price of each massage? You've got to use an iron fist.

And that, my friends, is what I mean by the "perverse incentives of capital." Most franchise owners and spa owners and chiropractors don't see an alternative to paying the minimum while extracting the maximum, even if it means the destruction of their own workplace culture. That's how you get rich in this industry. Indeed, it's the only way to get rich in this industry, so what's the alternative? If it means that every business you own eventually devolves into a morass of resentful employees and complaining customers, that's just something inherently wrong with massage therapy as a business.

You'd better hire stricter managers to keep everyone in line. Kindness and generosity? Not an option.

Being your own worst boss

You might be saying, "but Ian! I run my own business and I'm still feeling burned out!" If that's the case, I've got the sneaking suspicion that it's still your boss's fault.

Think about the expectations that you're putting on yourself and on your clients, and consider the demoralizing effects these can have when they're allowed to get in the way of your mission and values. I'll give some examples, but this isn't meant to be an exhaustive list. These are common practices in the industry, and as you look at how they can subvert a therapist's former enthusiasm for massage, try to use the same lens to look at your own practices and how they might be starving your internal flame of oxygen.

Always on call, never unavailable: I see this so often it might as well be an unwritten rule for self-employed massage therapists. They answer their business line at all hours (or don't have a separate business line and just give out their personal number), and their unofficial motto is, "I can fit you in." This tends to lead to utter schedule chaos as some days have eight appointments and others have two divided by a six-hour break, all based on making scheduling as convenient as possible for every client.

Competing for last place: This is the race to the bottom where you try to undercut the undercutters. Massage franchises charge $60? I can get away with $50, if I work more hours. People on Groupon are selling gift certificates for $40? I'll run a sale for $30. As long as people don't redeem them all at once, I can survive.

Relying on tips and upsales: Just like a bad boss will pay you a pittance because "you'll be making it up in tips and bonuses," this is something we do to ourselves with predictable consequences. Doing a huge Groupon campaign will garner you months of clients who want full value work for rock bottom prices. This can only be sustainable if you're able to extract more value from these clients, pushing add-ons and more deeply discounted services, and praying that this next person will actually tip.

Being everything to everyone: Only the worst boss would keep assigning you ultra-deep pressure clients when you've complained of wrist and thumb pain. So why is it that we keep accepting and trying to accommodate clients who are clearly looking for someone else's massage, and who keep pushing the outer limits of our physical capabilities? Why accept clients who push our ethical boundaries, or who are looking for a modality we're not trained in?

Expecting invincibility: We are only human, and we're made of living tissues with certain physical tolerances and physiological limits. A person can only run on guts and coffee for so long before body parts start complaining and the cerebral cortex checks out. Yes, you technically can do forty hours of massage per week, and some people do so without consequence, but what does *your* body need? Would a good boss give you a seventh massage at the end of an exhausting day?

That creeping sense of precarity

Why do we do this to ourselves? Why do we fall prey to the same sabotage that bad bosses inflict on their businesses? Well, here in the United States at least, we're working without a net. Getting and keeping healthcare can be tied to your ability to pay, as can your ability to keep your business space and housing. A bad month of income can mean utter crisis, with no unemployment insurance or other assistance to catch us if our footing falters. Every politician talks about "supporting small business," but they really mean people who already have money and are willing to set up shop in their state. Being an actual scrappy small service provider is, by design or by neglect, needlessly precarious.

The problem comes when we allow that sense of precarity to extend to every corner of our business culture and self-image, letting it override our values as massage therapists. When we approach clients and business from a place of insecurity, we tend to engage in grasping behavior that *inhibits* our growth rather than promoting it.

We also tell ourselves a story that just isn't true: "If I'm just perfect enough, and available enough, and willing to sacrifice enough, I'll finally be a worthy massage therapist."

The simple fact is that you're already worthy, and you were worthy with that very first stroke in your very first Swedish class. You're applying conscientious contact in a systematic way, and that is worthy. You're spending more continuous time with clients than anyone in any other healthcare modality, giving those clients the full spotlight of your attention, and that is worthy.

Worthy of what? Of compensation. Of professional regard. Of self-regard. Just ask any client who has finally discovered massage after decades of struggle with chronic pain — even if massage doesn't lead to full symptom resolution, it can represent a fundamental shift in how that client relates to their own body. Finally, an approach that doesn't just involve pills and shots and being waved away. An approach that isn't 10 minutes of attention followed by weeks of a seemingly arbitrary, assembly-line approach to rehabilitation (sorry, physical therapists, but a lot of you are stuck in factories too).

Once you realize the worth of massage therapy, a lot of the business strategies above stop making sense. Why would we compete with franchises and discount services in their race to the bottom? The message that this sends to clients is that our service is cheap and undifferentiated — they come in with low expectations and are primed to dismiss us and our work. It can be nice to blow these clients away rather than sinking to meet their expectations, but this usually ends with praise rather than a rich return. They leave marveling at what a bargain they've stumbled on, and eagerly await your next round of deep discounts.

Now, think about the message that this sends to you, in your heart of hearts. The progression is predictable: You start off by offering an hour of excellent massage for $40 because "I've got to pay my dues" and "I need to draw in clients." Elder therapists tell you that they suffered through that and worse, and smirk about kids barely out of massage school who think they can charge $80. You go through months of offering beautiful, golden massages for rock bottom prices. Each client who doesn't tip feels like a personal insult, and every client who disappears feels like a failure. As you internalize these perceived shortcomings and slights, you adjust your massage to meet your new valuation of yourself, and of clients, and of massage as a business. Resentment sets in, and you resolve to keep your best work for clients who actually value you.

The same when you make yourself always available, willing to make last minute changes that wreck your day, or that saddle you with an eight-hour shift that only has three half-hour sessions. Your clients perceive that you're a convenience, a trifle, and that their whims are what matter in this relationship. You implicitly tell yourself the story that your personal time is worthless, and so you're always ready to drop everything for clients, and you always feel like you're at work.

You're willing to put up with so much inconvenience and insult because, "if I don't, I'll lose this client. If I charge more, they'll leave." Even if you end up wildly busy because of these habits, you still feel like you're on the bubble, just on the edge of failure. You're not making a lot, your body hurts, your schedule is a mess, and you're so... burned... out.

Losing the layers

Over the course of this chapter, I've been implicitly inviting you to ask yourself a couple of questions: Is my work environment a drain on my morale? Has my view of myself or of my clients become twisted by the business decisions I've made, or the ones imposed upon me by my workplace? This can be a lot to unpack, but in doing so, you can start to reconnect with that excited massage student who couldn't wait to learn more about the hip flexors.

Let's start with your view of yourself. If you're feeling burned out, I'd like you to take an honest inventory of your career up to this point and find the factors that have sent the message that you are a *machine* rather than a person. It is this dehumanizing idea that underlies the burnout and attrition problems that we have in this industry. Franchises getting into bed with massage schools and slotting new graduates into a relentless assembly line, only to swap them out for a fresh graduate when each body fails. Chiropractors luring people in with decent hours and the promise of raises, only to ramp their schedule to the maximum while paying the minimum. Spas and clinics charging $110 per hour and passing $25 of that on to you, and then acting like they've done you a favor by paying more than a franchise. Independent therapists pushing themselves to the limit for the lowest prices in town, always on the precipice of failure, whether that be of their business or their body.

In all the above situations, there were numerous violations of the therapist's professional dignity, their authority as an expert, and their bodily autonomy. Being treated as a replaceable part is completely at odds with this truth: You bring something unique to the field of massage therapy. It is the light of your entire life's experiences shining through the lens of your training, creating a clinical approach and massage philosophy that is entirely your own. As physical therapist and teacher Walt Fritz says, you are not the sum of the modalities you have learned, you *are* the modality. Anyone trying to force you into a narrow box is depriving the world of something beautiful, something worth reclaiming.

Just as important as our self-view, I'd like us to consider how business decisions can change how we view our clients. In much the same way that a factory-like environment can be dehumanizing for you, it can lead to the gradual dehumanization of the very people you set out to help. This happens slowly and can be difficult to spot in real time: As your schedule is packed full and your body starts to fatigue and complain, it can be easy to see those clients as the source of your mental and physical distress. As you ponder the $20 that each hour-long session will net you, it's tempting to start discounting that human being just as steeply. You might start dividing your regulars and newcomers into easy and hard, tippers and cheapskates, "worth it" and "not worth it." This is the poisoned ground from which resentment grows.

Contrast this with how you related to each client back in massage school: New, impossibly complex, and maybe a little intimidating. Who knows what their body might be like, or the pain they might have? If they've had a lot of massage before, will I be able to meet their expectations? If this is their first ever massage, am I worthy to usher them into this world?

Over time your confidence grew, and you found the calm center within yourself that let you approach each new client, and all those questions, with less trepidation and more playfulness. You kept the curiosity and ditched most of the self-doubt, and you started having mastery experiences where clients would stand up with less pain, or request you specifically, or say, "you're the first person to ever find that spot." It was self-evident that each client deserved thorough consideration, not because of what they paid or how easy they were, but because they were a *person*. They embodied a full life's history, a world of philosophy and experience, and that embodiment was awesome to interact with. That consideration, and that awe, are something worth reclaiming.

Setting healthy business boundaries

We talked about boundaries with clients in chapter 6, so now let's talk about boundaries in business. Boundaries are how we define ourselves: What am I willing to tolerate from business partners and clients, and under what circumstances? What do I expect from others, and what do I do when they fail to meet reasonable expectations? Where do I end, and where does my business begin? By setting new boundaries, or simply making them firmer and more lucid, we can redefine how we see ourselves and our vocation.

I'll lay out my business boundaries, but these are just meant to be examples. Your boundaries will be based on your values and how you conceive of your business and its scope.

I expect to be treated as an expert in my field. I won't be rushed through a medical intake or agree to see someone without basic information — the prevention of medical errors is more important to me than making money or keeping a client. I have the right to turn down a session with someone who seems to be seeking work that I don't do, whether that be a modality I'm not trained in, techniques or pressure that cause me discomfort, or sex work.

I am the ultimate decision-maker when it comes to my own capabilities and my scope of practice. My client and I are the only ones that determine the treatment plan, except in cases where I'm working as part of a medical team (e.g., with a doctor or physical therapist). I won't be overruled by a franchise owner or a front desk associate when it comes to how I use my body, how I apply massage, or when I determine that massage is contraindicated.

My time is valuable. If a boss wants me to be on their premises rather than on my comfy couch at home, I expect to be paid. Not just as an optional add-on if I'm not getting enough hands-on hours; in addition to the hands-on hours! The same goes for workplaces that keep me on call for days when there *might* be clients. Either compensate me for being on retainer or expect me to be at the beach and unavailable.

The same goes for when I'm my own boss: I group my clients in tight bunches, and I don't accept an appointment five hours after another just to accommodate a client's needs that day. My availability is my availability, and I expect clients to plan ahead and make changes to find an opening, just as with any other healthcare professional.

I should be paid enough to allow me to retire one day. And afford healthcare. And afford time off, with a bit of travel. And heck, maybe start a family. This starts on the day I get my massage license. 600 bucks a week for a trained professional doing difficult and specialized labor is absurd, no matter how normalized it has become in the franchise world.

The same goes for when you work for yourself. You deserve good pay for hard work. When you're determining how much you want to charge, do so with retirement in mind. And emergencies. And leisure, for goodness' sake!

I am autonomous, and my consent matters. This is my overarching principle, the one that guides everything about my professional life. I think that a lot of burnout (and resentment, and workplace toxicity) starts when we lose sight of this idea and buy into the existing framework for how to be an employee, or how to build clientele: That we are somehow subordinate to the people with the money. That just because some guy has enough money to pay franchise fees, he's allowed to be a tyrant in his little patch of rented strip mall. That because we're asking clients to pay us, they're the ones who make the rules.

If you keep your autonomy in mind, it's much easier to stay above the fray in a crowded workplace where the norm is competition, gossip, and backbiting; you don't have to go along to get along. It's easier to say no to a company that expects you to sign a restrictive non-compete contract. It's easier to turn down clients who demand freebies or who expect you to come in on your day off. It's easier to say no when a client asks you to apply more pressure than your hands can comfortably provide.

This may seem adversarial at first glance: "I'm most important, so all must bend to my will!" But this is another instance of rebalancing a power differential, just like we do with clients. It's proclaiming, "I'm allowed to say no, and so are you." In a business relationship, just like in a personal relationship, both parties hold veto power at all times. Compromise is good, flexibility is good, but having a firm grasp of who you'd like to be as a massage professional can keep you from being slowly compressed into a corner and treated like a cog in a machine. Whether it's a boss doing this, or pressure that comes from within, it can be liberating to step back to your calm center and say, "no."

Building business on a firm foundation

Just as a creeping sense of precarity can cause you to engage in grasping behaviors that render your business less stable and effective, starting from a place of poise and self-assurance can set you up for long-term success. Not just that, it can allow for a serene environment, both in and out of the treatment room, that allows you to explore massage and all its many variations and related healthcare modalities, experimenting with your offerings and building your own identity as a therapist.

When I write about this, I find myself thinking of the psychological concept of *attachment*. This is an idea frequently cited when studying child development, but which also has implications across the lifespan. In this body of research, children with a *secure* sense of attachment to a parent or other caregiver will act in bold and experimental ways — they explore new spaces, they engage with others, and generally have lots of fun, knowing that their solid home base is always a glance away and ready to help. This secure attachment style develops when a caregiver is responsive to a child's needs, and available emotionally. Children with *insecure* attachment styles, those with frequent rejection experiences, will avoid new stimuli and hover near their caregiver, or withdraw from both caregiver and environment. If you're wondering whether this has implications for intimacy in adulthood, the answer found by research is a resounding yes.

But no matter your experience growing up, or in massage school, or in business since then: Each day is new, and you can be too. If you've found yourself adrift in a sea of self-doubt and negative self-talk, these are habits of the mind that can be changed over time. If you've been desperate to find your place in the business world and wound up changing yourself to suit some dumb boss, or to try to be everything to everyone, you can lay claim to a firm foundation based on a more stable sense of who you are as a massage therapist.

Imagine that you're a client in search of a good massage, and you've been disappointed by the rushed and lackluster offerings you've gotten at the local franchise. The therapists seemed frazzled, the massage felt like a cookie cutter routine, and you didn't really get a chance to explain what you needed. You've decided to look for an independent massage therapist, and you narrow your search to two candidates: One only charges 50 dollars, while the other charges a whopping 90 dollars. The former offers 20 different services, some of which are difficult to differentiate, while others have inscrutable names that mean nothing to you. That therapist seems to be available at all hours, with a post encouraging you to call for a same-day appointment, even offering a discount for that first session.

The latter therapist, on the other hand, isn't available until next week! They only offer three different services, which they explain clearly and at length. Their "about me" page lays out their training as well as their general approach to massage. They emphasize their ability to customize their sessions to suit different body types and comfort levels, and... well, you can't imagine this being rushed or cookie cutter. This person comes across as solid and professional, and they seem to radiate competence.

That's not to say that the more expensive therapist will be better at massage, or even able to give a superior session! A lot of excellent massage therapists wind up in that former category, compelled to compete in the race to the bottom. They've gotten caught up in making compromises which are likely to affect their output, as well as clients' perceptions of their value. Indeed, the hypothetical client above might try the cheaper session first, just for the sake of expediency, and find themselves going into the session with a skeptical eye and an expectation of low value.

Compare that to the client who takes the plunge, budgets the extra money, and plans ahead to see the full-price therapist. They're ready to get off the treadmill of discount sessions to see what massage can really do. Just by dint of paying more and having to go through some extra steps to schedule, they come into the office primed to be impressed. Because there was a higher barrier to entry, they did a little extra research on that therapist and their approach, and they're already on board, or at least curious and ready to learn more.

The secondary effects of security

Now, imagine yourself in the shoes of that second therapist. Rather than each day being rushed and unpredictable, you know your schedule a week in advance and can live your life accordingly. Rather than dealing with a lot of skeptics and bargain-hunters, you mostly see your regulars, along with a smattering of new clients who enter your office ready and willing to be convinced. Because you charge enough to live (and play, and retire!), you're able to limit your weekly output to something that's comfortable for your body, with plenty of time between sessions for recovery and client communication.

If the discount, always-available business is a storm with rapidly changing winds, the full-price business with a set schedule is a calm summer's day. Each setting tells a story to the client, and it tells a story to the massage therapist who lives that life.

My point here isn't that you have to charge a certain amount or conduct your business in the exact way that I do. My objective is to encourage you to make your business decisions mindfully, with *security* as your foundation rather than precarity. Just like a precarity mindset will lead to all sorts of self-sabotaging behaviors, a security mindset will have secondary effects of its own:

- You are free to set the schedule that suits you, rather than the one that suits the widest range of clients. Your time at work and your time off will feel like two distinct phenomena.
- You are free to give *your* massage rather than casting about for what's most crowd-pleasing or easiest to implement on a jam-packed day.
- You can present yourself however you wish rather than trying to appeal to everyone. You might feel drawn to a specialized niche, mostly working with post-surgical clients or triathletes or people who have migraines.
- You can turn down clients who are a poor fit, referring them to other massage therapists who have their own niche! That extra-deep-pressure client can go to your friend who loves to dig deep, and the client who wants myofascial work can go to your MFR buddy. They'll refer to you in turn, knowing that those clients will be in good hands.
- Following from that: You can act from a place of fellowship and mentorship rather than competition. Instead of being in a race to scoop up low-hanging fruit, you can band together with your fellow therapists to cultivate an educated client base who can each find their best fit.
- Finally, and most importantly, you can be more creative, experimental, and curious.

Let's focus on that last one. By finding your calm center and reconnecting with your values, you can have *more* fun, and *be weirder*. If you think that I've been describing a straitlaced massage clinic where strict business practices are more important than personal connection, then I've given you the wrong impression. By building on a firm foundation of positive self-regard and clear business boundaries, you are now free to branch out and explore. Just like a child with a secure attachment to their caregiver, by providing yourself with a firm foundation, you can feel free to range far and wide, knowing that there's always a stable home base to return to when you need to rest or retreat. You've got your high-quality client base, your regular schedule, your dependable and informed newcomers, and your colleagues in the massage and medical community. This is the fertile soil in which satisfaction can grow.

And even before you have all your ducks in a row, you can get out of the precarity mindset. Even if you're still at a massage franchise and are months away from being able to make your next move. Even if you've still got a hundred discount gift certificates outstanding and have jam-packed days for the next month. While you're in the process of forming a more secure foundation for your work, you can mentally step back from the frantic pace and condescending bosses and bargain-hunting clients, and you can choose who you want to be as a massage therapist. Realize that massage is a forgiving vocation, one where you can always create yourself anew from month to month. Even if it seems like you've dug yourself a deep hole with discounts and poorly defined boundaries, it's just a matter of putting one foot in front of the other and making your way toward daylight. As you do so, you'll pick up some clients who are perfect for you. As you toil in a franchise, you'll make lifelong friends among your co-workers, and convert some clients to true believers who will follow you wherever you go.

As you may have noticed, I'm asking you to have faith. Faith that you don't need to be perpetually available for every possible appointment. Faith that you can charge more than the bargain basement price that others around you have adopted and still have a full schedule. Faith that you don't need to compete with your fellow massage therapists, because there are plenty of clients, and you'll be the best fit for many of them. Faith that you can say "no" to unreasonable requests from bosses or clients and still survive in this industry; indeed, that doing so will net you higher quality bosses and clients in the long run. Start with small changes, both to your outlook and to your business practices, and I think you'll find that this faith is justified.

On alienation

When most people give advice about burnout, they do so with the assumption that, at its core, it's about boredom and stagnation. "Anybody would get burned out doing the same thing over and over! Try this slightly different thing!" This does work sometimes, and doing little things like changing your music or your room's layout can be refreshing, and can give us a peek out from under the blanket that's currently smothering our joy.

But that blanket isn't simple boredom — it's alienation. That feeling that "I don't understand how I ever enjoyed massage" isn't just a symptom of a bigger problem called burnout, it's the whole disease. I plan to belabor this point a bit, so bear with me. Alienation is a *loss of identity*. You no longer identify with the person you were when you started in this field, or who you were when you fell in love with someone. You've lost the person you were when you joined a religion, or started a club, or founded a non-profit.

Yes, these changes can happen because of growth. You might outgrow a relationship and realize you need a better fit for the new you, or you might find that an organization no longer fits your values as you unearth your internal philosophy. But alienation is distinct from growth in that it's about *erosion*. It's about contraction of self rather than expansion, often in a way that's directed by unconscious or external forces. It's why I spent the bulk of this chapter talking about the erosive forces of capital as an end unto itself — the sabotage that we press on ourselves and others when we equate success with wealth rather than connection and satisfaction.

This erosion can come from other places as well: A local bureaucracy that won't let you run your business without an endless procession of paperwork and fees. A month where three creepers wind up on your table and batter your hard-won sense of professional pride and safety. Bad business partners screwing you over, a landlord trapping you in a location that's suddenly the center of a construction zone, or even something small like a client writing a bad check. These indignities can add up over time, leaving you feeling alienated from the big ideas of massage, instead focusing on simply surviving the long slow barrage of disillusionment.

But, my friends, all that external junk that orbits around massage (and every caring profession) — that's the illusion. The jerks, the bad bosses, the predatory landlords. The need to hustle and sell and always be "on." These are all layers that obscure our relationship with our clients, and that can slowly make us lose sight of our former identity as a massage therapist. So, start by finding a more secure foundation and jettisoning all the external elements that are leeching you of your joy. Recognize the little blows to your dignity and take time to process them. And then, refresh your mindset.

What's new?

So far, we've mostly been talking about the big, apocalyptic type of burnout, that long slow loss of identity that makes you wonder why you ever got into this field. But every big burnout is preceded by lots of small burnout experiences — those days where going into work seems extra hard. Where clients get on your nerves for no good reason, and your co-workers could really stand to talk more quietly (or not at all). Your music sucks, your flow is off, and your next vacation feels like it's years away.

Dealing with big burnout means restructuring your business life and setting useful boundaries, but it also means shedding the baggage you've been accumulating during all those small burnout events. It would also be nice to have fewer of those bad days in the future, or at least be able to mitigate them when they occur, wouldn't it?

The main thing that bad days, bad moods, and burnout all have in common is a cynical state of mind. That feeling of having seen it all before — been there, done that, and it's not so great. It's the feeling of being stuck in a rut, and when you're stuck in a rut, you've got two options: New stuff, or new eyes.

New stuff is easy to implement, and this is usually what you see people prescribe when others describe burnout:

- **New music.** This one can be pretty big, because standard spa music is *dreadful.* Listening to that for long enough could drive anyone to a cynical worldview. My recommendation here is to find something that you enjoy moving to, or even something with a beat you can dance to. If you're leery of trying new music because you worry your clients won't like it, just ask! It turns out that clients enjoy good music too, and they might even have some suggestions.
- **New moves.** Or old moves that you'd forgotten about. If you find yourself in a rut, delivering the same massage routine day in and day out, it's time to try some different ways of approaching the body. This can even be arbitrary! Have yourself a Forearm Friday, where you spend at least ten minutes out of every session using your antebrachial region to make waves.
- **New sights.** Change your room around, or move your office across town. Seeing the same painting of a mountainside day after day can make you oddly resentful of that mountain. Try new colors, new lighting, and maybe keeping your blinds open a crack. One of the biggest precipitants of my bad mood days is being stuck in a room with no sense of the outside world.
- **New toys.** This one costs money, but it can be worth it. How about some new ways to apply heat to the body, like hot packs or tools that go in your hot towel cabinet? If you don't have a hot towel cabby, pick one up and start giving your clients miniature spa days. And while you're experimenting with new moves, why not snag a hydraulic table to help your body feel more comfortable? Try not to get addicted to new gadgets, but also... treat yourself.

"New eyes" is a tougher nut to crack. It means two things: Seeing through a beginner's eyes, and finding new perspectives. Each feeds into the other, and it can be a self-accelerating journey of discovery and renewal.

A fresh perspective

Start by reconnecting with your student self. Whether your school experience was a beautiful revelation or a frustrating slog, remember what it was like to encounter all those Latin words and kinesiological concepts for the first time. Remember your first time placing your hands on a practice partner's body, and the nervousness and anticipation that you felt. Whether you were a massage natural or not, remember how your hands eventually started to flow, and how all those complicated maneuvers started to become second nature.

When meditation teachers introduce the concept of beginner's eyes, they'll often ask new students to eat a raisin as if they've never encountered such a thing before. What is this unusual texture between my teeth? What are these scents and flavors, and what is my experience of savoring, then swallowing? This is often followed by taking a walk and observing the process like an alien on a new world in a new body. It's all disorienting by design, and the experience can leave you with a new appreciation for things you had been taking for granted. Tasting things is really cool, and wow, this planet is amazing!

So, think back to when you were first starting with massage, think about what it would be like to experience that process for the first time, and bring that newness into the here and now. No matter how long you've been practicing, really feel the connection as you conform your hand to the surface of a client's unique, incredible body. Allow yourself to feel awe at the internal structures as you glide over the surface. Be curious as you do so: What are these structures, and what do they mean to this client? What does this contact feel like to them?

This can take a lot of mental effort at first: Transporting yourself back in time to your student self, pretending to be an alien making first contact, putting yourself in your client's shoes. These can all be effortful forms of mindfulness, so don't be surprised if you find them fatiguing. My advice is to dip in and out of these new frames of mind, finding which ones feel comfortable for you, and with the full expectation that they'll become easier to access and maintain over time. And even when you're a pro at putting on those beginner's glasses, just realize that you don't need to live there – quick excursions to an alien world are all it takes, and they can serve as an excellent antidote to those days when you're feeling trapped in a dark room with an equally dark worldview.

Mindful massage can be a great daily tonic, but what are some big ways to shift your perspective?

Take a continuing education class. This one is obvious and is frequently recommended, but I'd like to tweak it a bit: Take a *weird* continuing education class. Take something that you'd never expect to use in your practice, really immerse yourself in it, and see if there's anything that you can import into your work. For instance, even if you never plan to give a massage using your feet, you could take an ashiatsu workshop and see what it has to offer you. What can your feet teach you about how to use your hands? What can the use of the overhead bars teach you about supporting yourself with your whole body as you work?

If you were to take a Thai massage or shiatsu class, what might you learn about rhythmic compression and pressure point work? The same with the multitude of energy work classes: Even if you're not on board with the theory behind them, they each have something special to bring to the world of bodywork. I never feel more connected to my client's nervous system than when I'm in my Polarity mindset, simply allowing my hands to connect two places with stillness or movement.

If you have the time and money, consider taking a *lot* of continuing education classes, both online and in person. These can act as vacations, they can connect you with your fellow practitioners who are on a similar journey, and they can refresh your perspective on massage in profound ways, even if you don't change a single thing about your routine.

Take more vacations. Again, a frequent recommendation, and for good reason. One cause of cynicism is monotony. If your weeks all look the same, eventually they start to *feel* the same, and it can seem like you're adrift from the timestream and stuck in a loop. Get yourself out of your massage room and out of your own head and go see some sights! This can be in conjunction with taking workshops as above, or just a full week traipsing in and around Yellowstone National Park. Want to make the whole "perceive like an alien" exercise feel easier? Go watch some buffalo while surrounded by bizarrely colored hot springs and the smell of sulfur. Go to Alaska and take a glacier cruise. If you're able, go see what this whole "Europe" thing is about.

Talk to a counselor. I want to recommend this for two reasons. First, a counselor (a licensed mental health counselor, psychologist, or social worker) can be an excellent resource for organizing your thoughts, figuring out the patterns in your life that aren't serving you, and getting into new habits that can refresh your perspective. I always have an easier time shaking myself out of stagnation when I've got a therapist rooting for me on a weekly basis, helping me figure out the little roadblocks I'm putting in my own way. Please know that you don't need to be at rock bottom to see a counselor, and they're pleased as punch to assist with professional and personal development.

The second reason is this: Burnout and depression have a lot in common, sometimes one masquerades as the other, and sometimes you're experiencing both. Here are the symptoms of depression, and stop me if you know this one:

- Loss of interest or enjoyment in previously pleasurable activities, a crappy state of affairs called *anhedonia*.
- Persistent low mood, meaning sadness, despair, or just a lack of positive emotion.
- Disordered sleep – too much, too little, low quality.
- Fatigue and low energy.
- Feelings of worthlessness; thoughts of self-harm or suicide.

Something that you might notice is that, if this constellation of symptoms seemed to be related to work, we would be quick to call it burnout! Loss of interest and passion, negative attitude, low energy and drive, questions about worth and meaning. Well well well, must be burnout, case closed. But no, if you find yourself regularly going into "funks," especially ones that persist for weeks at a time and that substantially affect your ability to live your life, then you seem to meet at least some of the criteria for a mood disorder[15]. Especially if you have thoughts about self-harm that creep in during those difficult times, it's worth seeking mental healthcare.

Before I move on from this point, I just want to make something clear: I get it. Depression and OCD go hand in hand, and I've struggled with months-long bouts of depression since I was a kid. It sucks, but there's good news: Just like depression creeps in, it eventually recedes, as dependably as the tides. Once I learned to have faith that I'd eventually emerge from any given depressive episode, it made each of them seem less dark and monolithic. More good news: Depression can be reduced in intensity and duration with lifestyle changes, mental habits, and specific strategies meant to counter its trajectory. In other words, no matter how big and immovable that wall of depression may seem, that's an illusion that depression itself creates. You have more power than you think, and the locus of control is yours to seize. And it's so, so much easier with professional help.

Cut back, or even quit. You might choose to reduce your massage hours and diversify how you make your money. If 30+ hours of massage per week is driving you crazy, you might really enjoy 15 hours of massage and a side gig. That's why I run my channel and teach; I can handle about 15 clients per week before my brain starts going dark and I start feeling bogged down.

Or, and this will seem a little counterintuitive for a book on massage, consider quitting and finding something that makes you happy! Because even if you implement all the strategies in this

---

[15] American Psychiatric Association. (2013). Diagnostic and statistical manual of mental disorders (5th ed.). https://doi.org/10.1176/appi.books.9780890425596

chapter, if you're far enough into the "pit of resentment" portion of disillusionment, you might find it difficult to make enough changes to dig your way out. If your alienation has become disgust, then do yourself a favor and get out from under that toxic stew as soon as possible. Retrain in a tech field, or another medical field. Any massage therapist would make an excellent physical therapist or PT assistant. Going to school for nursing or to be a physician assistant would be a good fit for someone with massage experience. There's esthetician school, hair styling, dental assistance and hygiene, and all manner of other paths that you might have been considering before massage school. If you're deep in the pit, it might be difficult to tell what thrills you, so this can be another job for talk therapy.

And if you do quit, just know that massage is always there. You'll always be a massage therapist to me. Even if it's just as a hobby or a part-time thing, it's a skill you'll always have, and a superpower that's always in your back pocket. One day, the big change of quitting might give you enough perspective to shake off the rust of alienation and help you remember what got you excited about massage in the first place. If that happens, then I hope you come back, and more than that, I hope you're able to structure your professional and personal life in such a way that massage can be a healthy and exciting part of who you are, rather than a long slow drag.

Away from dehumanization

Once you've determined that there's a problem and you've taken concrete steps toward pulling yourself out, how do you consolidate your gains and prevent that darkness from seeping in again? More importantly, how can you prevent new instances of burnout in the future? Do you have to constantly stay vigilant?

No, and in fact, once you recognize the pattern of feelings and behavior that comprise burnout, it's way harder for it to sneak up on you. A few years from now, if you feel that alienation from your work, and you notice that monotonous quality to your life, you can do a quick evaluation and fix the dehumanizing elements in your work environment. You can schedule a class and a vacation, switch up your music, and cut back excess hours. Rather than a constant game of whack-a-mole, you'll notice these trends as they arise rather than once they've become cemented and difficult to deal with.

But let's add on to that new power, and rather than just waiting for dehumanizing elements to creep into your work life (as they tend to do when money is involved), why not lean into *humanizing* elements that massage makes possible? In other words, what can massage offer you that makes you feel more connected, alive, and secure?

Moving from competition to collegiality: Alienation and isolation go hand-in-hand, and nothing is more isolating than feeling like you're in competition with your colleagues. Once you've realized that there are plenty of clients to go around, and more than enough work for everyone to be fully booked, why not flip that script and choose to opt out of competition altogether?

What I'm talking about here is something I call *mutual mentorship*. Rather than each of us hoarding our clients and our techniques like a dragon on a pile of gold, why not... do the exact opposite of that? Why not freely send clients where they'll best be served, with a spirit of love and acceptance as you do so? If a client gets "stolen away" by a better deal or a good sales pitch, why not wish that client robust healing and a good match? This goes beyond just non-attachment; it's actively saying, "I want my colleague to succeed, and I want my client to succeed, because that can bring us all satisfaction."

As for your massage secrets — who cares? Give 'em away! I've spent the last decade shoveling all my secrets out on YouTube like they're heaps of multiplying tribbles, and all that teaching has just led to me knowing *more*. Repackaging your thoughts and techniques in a way that makes them accessible to others is a form of creativity and transformation, and that process always leads to revelation. Every time I teach, I have little epiphanies that I can apply to my practice, which I can then teach!

I'm not saying to start a YouTube channel (though you could — there still aren't enough teachers and demo videos on there), I'm saying to be generous with your hard-won knowledge. Heck, be *promiscuous* with your knowledge. If you have a routine for working with sciatica symptoms that really does the trick, tell every massage therapist you meet. Offer to demonstrate it at your local AMTA meeting. Offer to demonstrate it the next time you have a massage therapist on the table. The same with business strategies: Share how you get your clients, offer to show people how to set up their Google ads, or help with a demo video.

I know this might seem scary, but all you're feeling is that old precarity mindset rearing its head. I invite you to have faith that sharing your secrets will just lead to more knowledge. Through teaching, yes, but also because generosity is contagious! You'll find that your colleagues are just as tired of miserly competitive practices as you are and will be more than willing to spill their secrets — and share their clients — once someone else gets the party started. Be like The Grateful Dead or Mystery Science Theater 3000 fandoms: Circulate the tapes, share generously, and build a community.

Making your work into play: Just like you can let go of competition, you can let go of massage as serious business. I've already talked about how being *really really invested* in your clients' recovery doesn't make that outcome more likely — and indeed, it can hinder their progress if it makes you engage in grasping behaviors, such as unnecessary escalation of intensity/invasiveness. What if we expanded that concept outward? What if we took everything about massage that makes it "serious" or "business" and just... let that go?

Think of the best massages you've ever gotten. For me, they were the off-work massage trades, given just for fun. They were the low-stakes sessions where we had both worked on each other so many times that half the duration was spent on experimentation, and any sense of routine was thrown out the window.

Now, think of the most enjoyable massages you've ever given. The ones that revitalized you and that got your brain churning with new ideas. Same situation, right? There's something special about that cauldron of creativity that comes with allowing yourself to play and experiment. It's a massive shift from that feeling of being locked into a routine so that you can give a new client the "perfect massage."

What if you just stopped doing that? Sure, keep your routine in the back of your mind. It's nice to have a solid foundation of techniques and sequences to build upon, or to fall back on when you'd like something reliable. But why not go on long massage tangents, and add some rocking and some forearm work, and try new ways of manipulating the leg, just because you feel like it?

"But Ian, will it still be an effective massage if I'm just sort of... screwing around?" This is another issue I'm going to ask you to have faith about, but yes. Not only yes, but heck yes. You can trust yourself to keep your client's needs in mind, and indeed, getting into this experimental headspace is one of the best ways of being responsive to the client's body as it actually exists. That's as opposed to trying to fit their body into a box, and trying to use techniques that don't serve them, or that don't quite fit the unique curves of their form. What if, instead, you let your communication lead the way? What if you followed your intuition?

Intuition is a funny word for me to use, because you never know what people mean when they say it. Is it a psychic thing? A spiritual one? An insight from your unconscious brain that springs into your mind without easily accessible reasoning? I prefer that last definition, but pick your poison. In any case, let yourself be led. Follow your intuition, even if it's not completely logical, and even if it doesn't show up on a pain referral chart or dermatome map. You'll find the most interesting things, like clients who feel a connection between their shoulder and their knee, or their hips and their neck. Why not make contact with both of those areas at once, acknowledging that connection and making it more explicit to the client's nervous system?

Be curious as you do so, and as you make every contact. What's going on in this client's low back, and how is it put together? What does pressure feel like here, and is it connected with their pain? You can ask some questions aloud while letting others be silent, just make sure to never lose that curiosity. Let it lead you too — allow yourself to be humble in the face of a new body on a new day, knowing that you can't possibly know everything about it. Maybe you can choose to act as if you know nothing.

As you cultivate this idea of a playful, intuitive, curious massage, realize that you're creating art. You're designing a session in real time, executing it with skill and grace, and at the end of it, you'll have delivered a massage that has never existed before and will never exist again. You're doing this not as an isolated artist in a lonely studio, but in active collaboration with a client, who is both canvas and co-creator. This is another instance of collegiality and community that can spring forth from massage; where once you might have felt alone, realize that you have a partner every time you create.

My little burnout

I have a confession to make. As I was writing this chapter, I had my first real case of writer's block. It's not that I ran out of ideas, but rather that I kept hitting dead-ends and writing about things that I didn't find compelling. All my ideas were bad, the book as a whole felt bad, and I wondered, why am I doing this?

But then it hit me. Wait a minute... that's burnout! You sneaky son of a gun, you almost had me. Once I had that information, I knew what to do next. I stepped away from the stuff that I found frustrating rather than forcing it. I spent some time playing in my book rather than working — I bounced around, adding here and there, just letting my intuition guide me. Once I felt like returning to this chapter, I did so with curiosity and without expectation. What happens if I write more today? What happens if I reread the chapter and sit with it for a while? What comes out if I brainstorm?

It's still not the perfect chapter, and it won't be a perfect book. But I'm hoping that my enthusiasm comes through, and my love for massage, massage therapists, and clients. I'd like the same thing for your work. If you let yourself be guided by a sense of security, and by curiosity, and by playfulness, what comes out? It won't be a perfect massage, but it can be better than perfect. It can be art.

Chapter 10: I Don't Know What Massage Does

This chapter will dip a toe into the most recent research so that you can have a good starting place when discussing what massage is capable of. Clients will ask: Can massage help with my pain? Can it help me recover from surgery, or from a marathon? Can it help with arthritis pain? These are questions that I want you to be able to answer with evidence in the back of your mind, even if you don't cite it directly. It's nice to be able to say, "yes, based on the most recent research, it's likely that massage will be able to help with your shoulder pain." It sounds smart because it is smart!

I also want you to be apprised of what massage has less of an effect on. For instance, we don't seem to be able to undo scoliosis or flat feet (something that I'm particularly bummed about). There's some evidence that we can help with migraines, but the effect size is usually rather small, and doesn't seem to outpace other treatments.

"But Ian, I've got a migraine client who has had almost complete resolution of her symptoms since she started massage!" And that brings me to the main thing I want you to take away from this chapter: Studies aren't real life, and averaged data will never tell the story of any one client. Here we're dealing with the *nomothetic* versus *idiographic* approaches to learning about our reality. These are two words that you're unlikely to ever hear again, but they stuck in my head during grad school, and now I'd like them to stick in yours.

A nomothetic[16] approach to studying the world seeks out general rules for how nature works – most relevant to our discussion, it looks at how humans generally respond to different treatments. In this paradigm we look at big representative samples of the population, apply similar treatments to all of them (often having a

---

[16] Nomothetic means "having to do with law," in this case the general laws of nature and biology. You can see the same base in the word "autonomous," which means "self-ruling." Bodily autonomy rules.

control group that receives a placebo), and average their responses together in hopes of finding what is useful and true. With this approach we often see rather small effect sizes for many treatments, even highly regarded ones that are considered the gold standard for care. We'll see that shoulder surgery for labrum repair has very similar outcomes to physical therapy, and that neither is radically more effective than simply waiting for the same length of time to pass. We'll see that massage is often only minimally more effective than a placebo, or that three very different approaches to massage are all equally effective.

Here's what I don't want you to take away from these big studies: "Well, I guess nothing works very well, and all massage is the same, so I'm mostly just spinning my wheels." No, these effect sizes are small because *that's the nature of nomothetic research.* By taking the results from a thousand different people and averaging them all together, we lump the miraculous recoveries together with the non-responders, and both of those are further smoothed out by all the people who only had a minimal response. We compare that to a control group who had the same passage of time, many of whom had a reasonable recovery as well (a phenomenon called *regression to the mean*).

We purposely take a big, noisy group of data, grind it into a digestible paste using statistical inference, and weigh that against similar groups to try to find a glimpse of which works better. This is unlikely to tell us what will work best for any individual person, and it tells us nothing about those miraculous recoveries (they may even get discarded from the data set!), but it sets us on the trail of a general truth about nature and how it works: "The effect size is small, but those who received massage had significantly less back pain than those who did not." Note: When you see the word "significant" in research papers, it means "probably not due to simple chance." It's a statistics thing.

Idiographic ("person-focused") research will tell a very different tale, and it will seem much more recognizable to those of us who work one-on-one with clients every day. Rather than condensing a thousand quantitative results down to their averages, we're plucking one person out of that sea of humanity and examining their story. There will be numbers to record and results to keep track of, but we're just as interested in the quality of their recovery as the numbers we can measure. This *qualitative* approach tells us about how that person perceives their body and the world, all without necessarily assigning a number to the finding.

The quality of relief

Consider someone with a chronic and persistent stiff neck problem, also known as cricks. They wake up about once per week completely unable to turn their head to one side, and they have considerable trouble sleeping the night after. This usually resolves soon enough, but it happens so often that it's making their life substantially worse. Here we've got some quantities we could measure: How frequently do you get a crick? How severe is the pain on a 1-10 scale? How many degrees of cervical rotation do you have compared to non-crick days? We've also got some qualities we could ask about: How is this affecting the quality of your life? How does it affect your mood? How is it affecting your sense of safety in your body, and control over your own destiny?

If this person were to come to my office, my expectation is that I'd be able to restore a good ten degrees of motion to their cervical rotation that day, and that they could expect better sleep that night. This is a fairly subtle result, quantitatively speaking, and one that might not show up in the results of a big trial where there were also non-responders and where there was less freedom to adapt the treatment to the client (more on this in a moment). In other words, the numbers would tell a rather unimpressive story.

But imagine what ten degrees of extra rotation *feels* like to someone with a locked-up neck. It feels like relief. It feels like being let out of a cage. It takes something that was absolute and hard and scary, and turns it into something softer and more yielding. They might still need to turn their torso to check their blind spot while driving, but there's less pain involved, and less frustration.

Think about this any time you see a small difference in a study on massage, or when you've got a client in your office who "isn't making much progress." Yes, they might still get back pain just as frequently, but they keep returning for a reason. Even if their stiff back is still reducing their range of motion by the same number of degrees, think about what it means for them to be pressing against that pain and being an active participant in their own recovery. Think about their experience of having someone manipulate that tissue without it being painful or scary, and how that can empower them to try some of their PT exercises with the same spirit. And even if the pain is still there, consider what it means to feel connected to their back rather than mentally cutting it off and throwing it away. It's no longer their "bad back," but a work in progress, a piece of a whole human on a journey of rehabilitation.

The idiographic advantage

There's something else that we can do when working with individuals that you won't see in any large study: We can adapt. We can tinker, and try far-out ideas, and run little experiments that might only last a minute apiece. Compare this to a large trial of massage that you might find in a medical journal: When trying to detect a real effect that is generalizable to the larger population, researchers *have* to be strict about what treatments are used and how. Every massage therapist treating that sample of people with similar low back pain needs to do the same routine, in the same order, with the prescribed level of intensity and duration for each arm of the study. If each therapist were allowed to freestyle or make up their own routine, the results would be rendered meaningless by the sheer inconsistency. Who's to say what caused the outcome?

The strictness and necessary homogeneity of nomothetic research can make a lot of useful healthcare approaches seem lackluster at a glance. People often claim that psychiatric medication is little better than placebo because trials of Prozac, for example, only show small effect sizes in large studies on depression. Once again, this is to be expected. The people with complete remission are being averaged with the non-responders, and both are being lumped in with those only having a middling response.

Now consider how this differs from the way that psychiatry operates in the real world: The psychiatrist doesn't simply prescribe a single medication and then throw her hands up in defeat when the response is poor. No, she'll track the patient's progress, and if their depression is persistent or recurrent, she'll try a second drug, or a combination. She might try transcranial magnetic stimulation, or psychedelic therapy, or even send the client to a meditation retreat. As this progresses, she'll have her patient see a counselor who she trusts to help that particular individual with their unique life situation, while also encouraging lifestyle changes that promote mental wellness, like aerobic exercise, yoga, massage, and so on. It's this adaptability and holism that makes a person-focused approach so powerful, and that also makes it hard to translate to well-controlled medical research.

Let me tell you about a client of mine who would have washed out of any study on back pain, but who found massage greatly helpful. She had persistent upper back and neck pain, and physical therapy and chiropractic treatment had either failed to help or had exacerbated her pain. I started with what I considered my standard pressure and routine, and sure enough, she experienced pain and spasm.

From there we adjusted rapidly and radically, decreasing the pressure to a tenth of my normal amount, and avoiding specific points that seemed to trigger spasm. Through weeks of experimentation, we found that she could tolerate more direct pressure to the area while supine, and that broad contacts with my forearms were useful while prone. Finally, by a stroke of intuition and luck, we found that she could receive direct, moderate pressure to the area while her shoulders were in a flexed position (i.e., her hands were resting on a stool near her head while prone). This approach provided the most durable pain relief between sessions, and she enjoyed finally being able to receive work in an area that had seemed rather sensitive and even scary previously. Over time we settled into a unique routine based on these findings, one that I've never used on anyone since.

This is the power of massage therapy as a discipline. As we discuss big studies and whether massage has an effect on any given condition, remember that we're not constrained by strict methodology, and that our clients will be individuals with endless potential for resilience and recovery. Use the studies to find the general direction of reality and how it works, and then use your intuition and adaptability to apply those principles in new and exciting ways.

A haphazard review of recent literature

This section will be somewhat random rather than comprehensive and methodical. It's meant to showcase research that represents what massage is capable of, with an emphasis on recent work and meta-analyses. My goal is for you to be conversant in the current state of massage research, and to feel more confident when talking to clients about what massage can do. I encourage you to follow the links in the footnotes and spend some time immersing yourself in these papers — each of them includes their own literature review full of useful information and citations, which you can follow to find even more. It's a rabbit hole that's worth going down!

As you do so, remember that research literature has its own language, and the only way to become fluent in it is to overcome that initial resistance to the dense and difficult prose. A lot of the words used are nearly unique to academic language, so there's no shame in consulting a medical dictionary or research glossary. You can also just let your eyes skip over the parts that seem to be nonsense and go straight to the meat: The method section (what they did) and the discussion (what the results mean). These usually contain the most comprehensible language, and they tell you what you need to know about what the research was, and what it demonstrated. As you do so, just keep an eye out for papers that seem to show something a little too extraordinary. Researchers are people like everyone else, and everyone wants to have a flashy new finding. Read with a skeptical eye and be tentative when you're relating new findings to clients. Try "new research seems to indicate this" rather than "they just proved that massage can make dogs live longer." (There's no paper that claims this, it's just something that I dearly want to be true)

Massage works: Let's just get this out of the way at the beginning: Massage is effective for pain reduction, and lots of research says so. For this I'm happy to just look at recent meta-analyses and note that massage came out on top most of the time. If you're not familiar with the term meta-analysis, it's a study that studies other studies. They take all the data from the smaller studies, process them into new data that can be directly compared as if all the participants were part of the same pool, and then look for differences among treatment groups and control groups. It tries to make something clean and comprehensible out of something *very* messy — massage research is just as heterogeneous as massage as a field — and it's a process that magnifies the nomothetic research problem that I wrote about above. If this average of averages can detect even small differences between two approaches, I'm reasonably confident that there's a real effect being found. The differences might seem slim when you dig into the results section, but remember that these averages are masking a wide range of outcomes, some of which were life-changing for the individuals involved.

To start, let's look at a 2016 meta-analysis of massage for pain populations by Crawford et al.[17] (et alia, shortened to et al., roughly means "and the rest"). They found 32 studies on massage for pain that met their inclusion standards and compared the average amount of change. In other words, no matter what test the individual research teams ran, they just asked, "how big was the effect compared to pre-treatment?" The included studies compared massage to no treatment, to active treatment (spinal manipulation, traction, splinting, and others), and sometimes to a sham treatment specifically designed to seem active while doing nothing. They found that massage was considerably more effective than no treatment, that it was somewhat better than sham treatments, and it held its own against the other active treatments without being the runaway victor. It varied from study to study, with some showing very little effect of massage and

---

[17] https://www.ncbi.nlm.nih.gov/pmc/articles/PMC4925170/

others declaring it clearly superior, but after all the averaging and statistics, massage was shown to be effective for pain. If a meta-analysis comes to that conclusion, I'm satisfied.

Massage for low back pain: Furlan et al.[18] (2015) looked at the outcomes of 25 trials involving massage and low back pain. They found massage to be effective for short-term pain reduction when dealing with chronic low back pain, but not for long-term reduction. Massage compared favorably to passive and active control groups. Despite this, Furlan et al. delivered the devastating sentence, "We have very little confidence that massage is an effective treatment for LBP." This seems to be from the inconsistency of the outcomes (massage didn't always help with function, even when it helped with pain), and the general heterogeneity and poor quality of the studies involved. These are common themes when looking at studies of low back pain, by the way: The research is messy, there are rarely definitive outcomes, and everything seems to help *a little*. When everything seems kind of effective, it's easy to conclude that nothing is actually helping. I tend to think that this is a job for an idiographic approach that adapts to each individual. Onward!

Massage for shoulder pain: Yeun[19] (2017) analyzed 15 studies on massage and shoulder pain, and found fairly substantial improvements in the short-term, with smaller improvements maintained over the long term. While most of the included studies compared massage to an inactive control group, the comparisons to active treatment groups were similarly robust.

Massage for neck pain: Kong et al.[20] (2013) did a meta-analysis and systematic review of massage for neck and shoulder pain, but I'll focus on the results for the neck. They found that massage was considerably more effective for pain relief than an inactive control group (e.g., being on a waiting list), while it was comparable to other active therapies such as exercise and traction.

---

[18] https://pubmed.ncbi.nlm.nih.gov/26329399/
[19] https://www.ncbi.nlm.nih.gov/pmc/articles/PMC5462703/
[20] https://www.ncbi.nlm.nih.gov/pmc/articles/PMC3600270/

I invite you to delve into this paper a bit. One interesting study is a comparison of acupuncture and massage by Irnich et al.[21] (2001). On a pain scale of 0-100, acupuncture was approximately twice as effective as massage for neck pain relief, bringing participants from an average of about 50 down to about 25! That's a huge reduction, and it certainly has real-world significance. Of interest is their implementation of massage, which is described as follows: "Techniques included effleurage, petrissage, friction, tapotement, and vibration. Mode and intensity were chosen by the physiotherapist [...]". Is that how you would treat neck pain? Indeed, some of those techniques seem contraindicated in this scenario. Just your regular reminder to dig deeper than the title and abstract when reading research about massage — are they talking about a form of massage that maps onto your approach, or that even represents best practices?

Something else to note is that these researchers found no significant difference between acupuncture — in this case, needling of points in accordance with traditional Chinese medicine as well as dry needling of trigger points — and the use of an inactivated laser pen. While there was a trend toward active acupuncture being more effective, the sham treatment still had an awesome showing, often reducing pain by nearly as much. This is similar to other studies that compare active and sham acupuncture[22]. Is the lesson to throw acupuncture out the window? No, we just saw that it can be really effective! The lesson here is to respect the power of placebos, and that certain placebos can be quite potent indeed.

Massage for migraine: A review by Chaibi et al.[23] (2011) included a whopping two studies comparing massage to a group receiving no treatment; in both studies, migraine sufferers experienced clinically significant reductions in symptoms, both during the treatment period and afterward. One study found a reduction in intensity, while the other found a reduction in frequency with no change in intensity. Go figure.

---

[21] https://www.ncbi.nlm.nih.gov/pmc/articles/PMC33515/
[22] https://pubmed.ncbi.nlm.nih.gov/26707074/
[23] https://www.ncbi.nlm.nih.gov/pmc/articles/PMC3072494/

One reason I mention the Chaibi review is that, when examining the use of physical therapy for migraine, the study they included (yes, just one study — non-pharmaceutical approaches to migraine are rarely examined) showed worse outcomes for the group receiving physical therapy than for a relaxation group. But then, they *switched* approaches, offering the relaxation group physical therapy and vice versa. When they did this switcheroo, they found that half of the participants who had not improved previously experienced significant improvements from the other approach! So, an interesting lesson: It turns out that trying a bunch of approaches can help a lot of non-responders. If they'd had a third or even a fourth approach up their sleeves, maybe they could have gotten that number up even higher.

Massage for arthritis: For osteoarthritis, massage shows fairly consistent benefits for pain management. For example, in a rather large and well-controlled study on knee osteoarthritis, Perlman et al.[24] (2018) found that eight weeks of weekly Swedish massage reduced participants' pain, stiffness, and dysfunction significantly more than treatment as usual or a light touch protocol. Following this with twice-monthly massages maintained these results, but it wasn't significantly better than switching them to light touch or usual treatment. The lesson here? A high-frequency protocol of massage (even good old Swedish!) can be great for knocking out some pain and dysfunction in knee osteoarthritis, which can then be maintained by their doctor's usual treatments. What a great add-on! It makes me wonder if a longer protocol of weekly massages might have accomplished even more.

There have been positive findings for rheumatoid arthritis as well, but the sample sizes have been too small for me to consider it definitive. In any case, *something* seems to be happening to people with joint degeneration, simply from receiving massage in the general area. This is an important finding! It shows that, while we can't affect the joint space or reverse cartilage loss, we can still reduce pain and increase function. In any case of chronic pain, there are multiple

---

[24] https://www.ncbi.nlm.nih.gov/pmc/articles/PMC6420526/

contributing factors, and we can help soothe the nervous system and reduce sensitivity. That can be a big deal.

Massage for fibromyalgia: Li et al.[25] (2014) examined 9 studies on the effect of massage on patients living with fibromyalgia, finding that massage protocols lasting longer than five weeks were associated with somewhat modest improvements in pain, anxiety, and depression. There was a positive trend for sleep quality, but it did not reach statistical significance. An interesting outlier in this study was the inclusion of Ekici et al.[26] (2009), which Li counted as a negative result. The reason is that the "massage" group (connective tissue therapy, which is similar to Rolfing), was outperformed by the "active control" group, which was manual lymphatic drainage. Both of these are massage! A good reminder to dive into the data when you're reading a study, and to possibly consider brushing up on your MLD skills when you're working with clients with fibromyalgia.

Speaking of a massage vs. massage battle royale, which modality is the best for fibromyalgia symptoms? That was the question researched by Yuan et al.[27] (2015), using 10 studies to compare different approaches. This rather small meta-analysis showed a robust effect from myofascial release, with smaller (but positive!) effects from MLD, connective tissue therapy, and shiatsu. Swedish massage did not appear to have any positive effects. Again, this is a small study made up of small studies, so don't change your life based on it — but consider myofascial (within your client's comfort level!) and/or MLD for your clients with fibromyalgia.

Massage for general wellness: This will be the most haphazard part of my review of massage research, because there are a lot of studies that show these effects, but little attempt has been made to synthesize the results. So instead, let's look at random papers that I feel are important!

---

[25] https://pubmed.ncbi.nlm.nih.gov/24586677/
[26] https://pubmed.ncbi.nlm.nih.gov/19243724/
[27] https://pubmed.ncbi.nlm.nih.gov/25457196/

Let's start with a paper by Nerbass et al. [28] (2010) that examined the use of three consecutive nights of back, shoulder, and neck massage for patients directly following cardiac surgery. While there was some evidence of pain reduction, the big finding was more effective sleep at night and less fatigue during the day. That sounds pretty great right after a major surgery. Pinar and Afsar[29] (2015) tried a week-long protocol of nightly 15-minute massages for caregivers of family members with cancer, and they found a strong reduction in anxiety, cortisol, blood pressure, and heart rate. The caregivers slept better too. Unal and Akpinar[30] (2016) offered twice-weekly foot and back massages to hemodialysis patients for four weeks, finding a substantial reduction in fatigue and increase in sleep quality. Foot massage came out ahead, by the way. Karaduman and Çevik[31] (2021) examined sacral massage *during* labor, finding that the participants who received this treatment reported significantly less anxiety and pain. Finally, Rapaport et al.[32] (2021) looked at twice weekly Swedish massage for twelve participants with generalized anxiety disorder. They noted a huge drop in symptom scores over the first six weeks, with a more modest trend in the right direction in the following six. This study is small, preliminary, and has no control group — but with all those huge caveats, this is a pretty stunning finding. I look forward to a larger, well-controlled follow-up.

What are you supposed to do with these vastly different protocols used on wildly different populations? I'm hoping you'll get a sense of how even little doses of massage can make people feel better. Less stress, better sleep, less fatigue, even in difficult life circumstances. There are multitudes of these studies, often with the results about mental state and sleep being secondary to results about pain. In other words, you have to dig into the literature to get a sense of just how much massage can affect wellbeing. While the research is

---

[28] https://www.ncbi.nlm.nih.gov/pmc/articles/PMC2999703/
[29] https://pubmed.ncbi.nlm.nih.gov/26745049/
[30] https://pubmed.ncbi.nlm.nih.gov/27502815/
[31] https://pubmed.ncbi.nlm.nih.gov/31298494/
[32] https://www.sciencedirect.com/science/article/pii/S0965229920318604

still in its infancy, I'm confident in recommending massage therapy for clients with anxiety, poor sleep, and other problems that relate to quality of life.

How often should people get massage? The consensus among researchers seems to be once or twice a week, at least for an initial period of eight-ish weeks. In the Perlman paper above, the researchers found that a twice per month regimen was effective for maintaining results, but without any obvious additional pain reduction. Another paper led by Perlman[33] (2012) compared twice-weekly to once-weekly massage, and found that once per week was just as effective for knee osteoarthritis symptoms. That's great news! It's a much easier sales pitch to make, and it's more convenient for clients to fit into their lives. Oh, and they found that 30-minute sessions were not as effective as 60-minute sessions, even when total time per week was equal. I'd love to see a follow-up with 90-minute sessions, but for now I feel pretty good about my decision to take short sessions off my menu. Your mileage may vary.

How to recognize a reasonable claim

I was thinking of writing a section on how to recognize good research, but that part is pretty simple:

1. Look for a large sample size. More than 50 participants is impressive for massage research, but fewer than that can still produce useful data. Think of these smaller studies as possible leads for your practice, and good candidates for replication in larger studies in the future.
2. Look for an active control group. The non-massage group should be something other than a bunch of poor sods left on a waiting list. They should receive some sort of treatment that makes them think, "hey, maybe I'm in the active wing of this study, and maybe this will make me feel better." Examples of this are sham ultrasound treatments, or sham trigger point

33 https://pubmed.ncbi.nlm.nih.gov/22347369/

treatments that use random points. It's difficult to give a placebo massage, but the researcher should at least try.

3. Look for blinding. A good study should have researchers *and* participants who don't know whether they're in the active intervention group (the "real" group) or the control group. This is called double blinding, and its purpose is to avoid bias in both researcher and participant. It's also extremely rare in massage research. If they can achieve even partial blinding, it's a sign of a higher quality study.
4. Look for claims that follow the results. If the outcome of the active group and the control group were similar, be dubious of any researcher who claims to have made a breakthrough.

As you dive into research on a regular basis and become more fluent in its dense language, it becomes easier to separate the high-quality studies from the ones that should be set aside into the "might be relevant one day" pile. Look for researchers who recognize the limitations of their study, especially as they relate to the markers of quality listed above, such as proper blinding. Look for researchers who are tentative about their conclusions, and follow their lead. Massage is an old art but a young science, and it's wise to present our results and our expectations with some humility.

But what about claims that aren't part of research? How can you recognize when continuing education providers are giving you good information versus when they're blowing hot air? When your teachers are telling you about the body, how can you separate the indisputable facts (e.g., "the glomerulus is the functional unit of the kidney") from the unsupported claims (e.g. "this point on the foot is related to the kidney")?

Well, you could spend the rest of your life shouting, "but where does it say this in the research?!" Shout it loudly and often, and you'll sound like the most intelligent person in any given room. You'll also have very few massage techniques at your disposal, and you'll have trouble learning from the hard-won clinical experience of your peers and teachers. It's wise to be led by research and tempered by skepticism, but being dogmatic about it is a good way to miss out on nuance, and on all sorts of interesting approaches born of personal experience. I can't cite a study when I tell you that rocking the sacrum is amazing and useful, but you'd be missing out if you just dismissed it out of hand.

To identify a reasonable claim, look for these qualities:

1. There is a clear cause and effect relationship. When you compress certain points on the upper traps, many people will feel referral in the base of the skull. When you apply 10 minutes of Swedish massage to the upper back, the muscles will usually feel softer and warmer.
2. The claim is tentative and acknowledges variations in human physiology. I'm much more likely to believe a teacher who says, "this works about half the time" than one who claims to have something that works across the board.
3. The claim doesn't rely on a sales pitch. If a continuing education teacher is demonstrating an amazing technique to erase pain, ask yourself, "would this still work without all the explanation? Would it work in a one-on-one environment without all the social pressure of a classroom?"
4. The claim doesn't rely on frequent tests and retests. Frequent retesting can make any treatment seem effective, mostly because clients will try to help by nudging the outcome in the direction that the tester seems to want (in the world of experimental psychology they call these *expectancy effects*).

There are many claims swirling around the realm of massage that are both unproven and unprovable, so my recommendation is to consider them toys to add to your toy box rather than becoming overly attached to a foundational theory or approach. I don't have much faith that the theory underlying reflexology would survive close scrutiny by a research team, but... reflexology is still great! It's a completely unique way of dealing with the foot, and it reliably creates relaxation effects (and even altered states) that don't happen when working with the foot in other ways. It's cool, and there's a reason that it has stood the test of time, even if we're not affecting the internal organs or their function.

But what if it's just a placebo?

Indeed, what if all of massage is just a particularly powerful placebo that outpaces other placebos?

First, I think this question is missing the point. It reminds me of the debate around climate change: What if the scientists are wrong and it's not man-made? Okay, fine. Why not just make the world a less polluted and more livable place anyway? Why even fight about fossil fuels when we could just stop burning them as soon as possible, which would have a million positive effects?

If massage is a placebo, so what? It's a darn pleasant one if so. Maybe the outcomes that people have are "all in their head," but how is that an argument against massage as a modality? If we've found a useful lever for manipulating the brain and how it relates to the body, why not use it? Especially one that feels good, and that creates a sense of connection and wholeness.

Second, placebo isn't a dirty word, and it doesn't mean "fake." Another term for placebo is "nonspecific treatment effect." These are the secondary effects that surround being in a therapeutic environment, or that stem from the feeling of being treated. Just going to the doctor and having your lymph nodes palpated can be enough to reduce your health-related anxiety and give you a feeling of wellbeing. Just being in the soothing space created by your psychologist can do half the work for them, representing a refuge that you get to escape to once per week. How much of the health outcomes are from these incidental factors rather than directly from a medication given, or the psychological modality used?

Does it matter? These are real effects, and they're worth pursuing. A psychologist wouldn't make their space stark and uninviting just to isolate the "real" treatment effects. That might be worthwhile for a study, but I want to harness every tool at my disposal to help my clients feel better. If that means having salt lamps and a singing bowl in my room, even if they only create nonspecific treatment effects rather than directly affecting the body, then I'll happily make my room cozier and more therapeutic.

Third, I'm more than happy to help people find a placebo that works for them. I don't think that spinal manipulation accomplishes much directly, and I consider the "subluxation theory" that underlies it dubious and outdated. But I do think that it's a powerful placebo. It's so *crunchy* and dramatic, and there is that hit of adrenaline and endorphins afterward that makes it feel like something big and momentous just happened. If someone tells me that a chiropractor knocked out their neck pain, would I just say, "nuh uh"? No, I'd be happy that they found something that worked for them! The same for acupuncture, or magnetic bracelets, or the power of positive thinking. If someone finds a piece that slots neatly into the puzzle of their life, then I'm just happy they found it. Even if massage is just a powerful placebo, it has helped countless people, it outpaces other treatments in many scenarios, and I'm glad to provide it, regardless of how it achieves its effects.

Finally... I don't think it's just a placebo. I think that the placebo effect is involved (i.e., that we're influencing the mind as we work on the body, and that the environment we create helps this process), but massage is simply too powerful and unusual a stimulus to have no specific effects on the body. No other healthcare modality works with the body in a way that *feels good* for extended periods of time. No other modality distorts the tissue in the same way that we do, or for the same duration. Massage produces delayed onset muscle soreness like a workout, it makes you feel high like a good jog, and it makes you sleep like a day at the beach. I think it's powerful medicine.

Is massage worth the money?

In other words, can we justify a chronic pain patient spending a thousand dollars over the course of two months for something with a pain reduction profile similar to yoga or physical therapy? I follow a number of physical therapists on Twitter who seem pretty emphatic that, no, manual therapy is not a good cost-for-time proposition, especially when you can just spend five minutes with the patient and have them do a bunch of strength training while overseen by an assistant (that last part might be me editorializing).

And it's true, massage does require 100% of the therapist's attention for the full duration, and it's time-consuming for both parties. Because of this, it's also more expensive on a per-patient basis, with those 5-minute consults or 5-minute spinal manipulations being much cheaper to administer, and much more lucrative per hour. Why would anyone be crazy enough to spend a full hour with a patient?

Because we don't have to apply the logic of capitalism to healthcare. We don't have to maximize profit and cut "waste," when that extra time and effort might mean another 5% reduction in the client's symptomology. For someone with chronic pain, 5% can be huge. If it can be achieved by adding a low-risk and potentially high-reward approach to pain to their regimen, why wouldn't we do so?

Because massage can *save* money. Many invasive and expensive treatments for pain (e.g., surgery for a labrum tear) can be avoided with noninvasive treatment, of which massage can be an important part. With massage acting as an analgesic, and even having effects on range-of-motion and daily function, it can be an important adjunct to physical therapy in rehabilitating a shoulder with a structural problem. This can avoid surgery along with the opioid prescription that often follows it, making massage an excellent proposition for avoiding time lost to convalescence.

Because massage can succeed where other treatments fail. This isn't something that I can cite a study for — again, a nomothetic approach is about prescribing a single standardized treatment, and it's rare indeed for a study to build in adaptation — but it's something that I've seen countless times in my clinical experience. Clients will sometimes come in with years of physical therapy and even surgery under their belt and find that massage is the key that finally frees them from their pain. I've seen this with TMJ problems, neck problems, low back pain, and all manner of hand and foot problems that people had accepted as part of their new life. "I guess I don't get to use this hand for anything." It turns out they just needed someone to pay attention to their shoulder and their wrist flexors and extensors, and suddenly they get a useful amount of their grip strength back.

And, because people are worth it. They're worth that entire hour of sustained attention and care. They're worth being lavished with kindness and compassion. Their pain is important, and their wellness is paramount. This is about more than just getting people functional so that they can return to work — this is about helping them feel safe and secure in their own body. Massage can empower people to take an active role in their own wellness journey, encouraging them to be proactive and to take back their locus of control. It can invite people to reconnect with the body that they had once rejected. What could be more worthwhile than that?

Interlude: Massage Myths

Fascia can be lengthened and unglued. I've talked about my qualms with a structural approach to pain and dysfunction a few times in this book so far, and it all comes down to this: Can we lengthen connective tissue in a lasting way? Can we break up adhesions?

The answer is "probably not," not without a scalpel. Connective tissue is composed primarily of collagen, a protein specialized for strength. Indeed, it's much stronger than the circulatory, nervous, and muscular tissue around it. For the omnivores in the audience, imagine taking a raw cut of meat and pulling it into pieces — which pieces fray apart, and which remain fully intact? The dense, collagenous tendons, aponeuroses, and coverings are all much more durable than mere muscle.

The same goes for adhesions and scar tissue — if two structures are glued together in the body, that "glue" is a net of collagen fibers! This leaves aside the issue of whether adhesions are even palpable in most cases. Why would we expect a thin net of fibers between two fascial layers to feel like much of anything? As you consider this, it's important to remember that these are living tissues invested with blood supply and nerve endings. Even if you could "break up an adhesion," the result would be internal bleeding and intense pain.

In the end, these are macroscopic, mechanical principles mistakenly being applied to a living, microscopic environment. All talk of "breaking up" or "stripping out" needs to keep this in mind: We're dealing with painstakingly deposited proteins being maintained by local cells, all supplied with hydration and nutrition by circulation and diffusion. Even if we could break that up, why would we? It would be so needlessly disruptive, especially when there's an easier way built right in.

If an area is riddled with scar tissue, what can you and your client do if you can't "break it up"? You can communicate with the local cells that maintain it. By mobilizing scar tissue and regularly deforming it, you can increase the activity of the local fibroblasts and white blood cells that are capable of remodeling it. By massaging the surrounding muscles and having your client use that part of the body in new and interesting ways, we can send a powerful signal that the body needs functional healing rather than just fast healing. While this is most applicable in the months following an injury or surgery, even mature scar tissue goes through changes over time. Functional healing is something that we can help promote, even if we can't do it in a single session.

"I need to work out your knots." Much of this follows from the myth above, but there's something that I want to highlight here: How sure can we be that a knot is a knot? What on Earth *is* a knot in this paradigm?

My working theory is that many massage students heard about knots and working them out in their education, or even from popular conceptions of massage and how it works. Others probably picked it up from their clients, some of whom love talking about how their last therapist found "so many knots," or "the worst knots they'd ever felt." We're then graded by how well we work with these knots, and knot-busting is seen as the highest form of massage.

But what is a knot? I'm sorry if I sound like a broken mp3 here, but it seems to me that the knot concept always precedes any sort of operational definition of the word, existing as a nebulous, self-defining and self-justifying entity, completely unmoored from medical classification. "I know it's a knot because I felt it, and when I busted it up, the client felt better."

And indeed, I'm sure fine work was done, and the client did feel better. All I ask is that, when we notice these patterns of cause and effect, or when we come up with mental models of what's going on in the body and how massage works, that we be skeptical of our own conclusions. When you notice that "when I do this, it helps with that," I'd like you to file it under "Possibly Useful Connection — Needs More Data."

Why? Because it's easy to accumulate superstitions in this field, or in any one-on-one caring profession. We see many people in pain, most of whom recover while they're under our care. We see many people have amazing experiences on the table, or report improvements to their life while they've been seeing us. And yes, I am convinced that massage can have broad-ranging effects on pain and mood and life, but I'm also certain that I'm only *partly* responsible for the changes in my client, and I only have so much control over the situation. Most clients will recover from pain with or without treatment (this is a phenomenon called *regression to the mean*, and it's why good studies have control groups). I imagine some clients would have epiphanies and sudden recoveries no matter who was working on them, and no matter the modality, just because they were ready. I do think that my current way of working is effective, and possibly more effective than other approaches, but I've got to have the humility to recognize that I'll never be able to compare each of my clients with their alternate reality twin who received a different treatment.

Yes, you perceived a tissue difference, and yes, the client responded positively to work there. But are there alternative explanations that should be considered? For instance, I find that when massage therapists tell me, "Wow, you have such a big knot," they're almost invariably pressing on the tendinous insertion of the levator scapulae muscle on the superior angle of my scapula. It's a big, bulky, twangy tendon. And no, it's not a knot, and it's not something that can be "busted up," no matter how ardently some massage therapists have tried. The same with various bumpy parts of the trapezius, which is a 3-dimensional muscle with many variations in texture and geometry. Please don't try to erase the part of my trapezius just medial to the spine of the scapula. I need that.

"But Ian, why does it work to bust up those knots?" Does it? The thing about the not-knots I mentioned above is that it can feel good to work on them, and they can be sensitive. Indeed, working on them long enough can desensitize them, at least temporarily, and it can reduce the overall tone in the area. You might also create some inflammation that makes the whole area feel turgid and homogeneous. So, you end up with something less crunchy and sensitive and more flabby and tender, and you and the client count that as a victory over that knot. But the knots always return, don't they? In fact, I'm betting the client suffers considerably the next day, and the knot might be even more sensitive the next time you see them!

I won't belabor this point further, other than to say: We don't need "knots." We don't need a big, obvious culprit for pain when there are a lot of complex, subtle explanations that deserve examination. We don't need to plant the idea in our clients' heads that they have a mysterious muscle problem that only massage therapists can identify and treat. We don't need to stigmatize normal anatomical features, even if clients wear their "most knots ever" badge with pride. Others will take that same information, worry about it endlessly, and carry it with them from therapist to therapist, hoping to find one who can finally solve their knot problem once and for all. I hope that you, faithful reader, are able to give them a better explanation, even if it's not nearly so definite as the one offered by the knot salesmen.

Massage is detoxifying. This is another one that seems to emerge from a logical dead end: "They had a detox response following their massage, so massage must be detoxifying." Ah, what's a detox response again? "It's where you feel unwell following an event where toxins are liberated into the bloodstream. It can be mild like a light hangover, or severe like a flu."

Oh, you're describing systemic inflammation! While some toxins might have that effect, that sounds a lot like someone had tissue damage and is now dealing with the consequences. How did you induce this detox event again? "I did extremely aggressive massage for a full hour."

Cue me screaming and running from room to room like Kevin in Home Alone.

I don't mean to be too hard on people who believe massage myths — there are lots of myths and superstitions in our profession, and most of them are harmless and well-meaning. Any profession that consists of daily single-participant experiments will find itself brimming with beliefs based on false pattern recognition, just from seeing B follow A more than once. If you notice that pressing on teres minor precedes a hip release, and then you repeat that trial and notice the same effect, you might come to the belief that the two are powerfully connected. It's false, and it doesn't follow any sort of internal logic, but it's harmless.

The "detox response" myth is harmful, because it takes something that is within the control of the massage therapist — the intensity of the session — and blames the outcome on the client. "That's just how some bodies respond," or "you should have drunk more water, like I said." It's finger-pointing, and worse, it's pathologizing. These therapists are telling clients that their body has a problem that only massage can reveal or treat, so not only is your pain a good thing, but you'd better come in more often.

And it all seems disconnected from a reasonable and testable question: Can massage release and remove toxins? This isn't something that there's research on, so I will be tentative in my conclusions. I see no reason to believe that massage is any more detoxifying than any other event that deforms tissue, such as a walk around the block or a dozen sit-ups. Even techniques that directly target the lymphatic system can only speed the return of lymph to the bloodstream; it's a faster version of something that was already happening. While these modalities might be able to accomplish cool and potentially useful effects like reducing lymphedema in a limb, these are temporary outcomes that represent a change in circulation *rate* rather than "finally clearing out that lymph."

In the end, this all seems to come down to a "stagnant blood" myth. There's a belief that there's bad blood hanging around in areas, often blamed on adhesions or knots, and the only way to clear it out is massage. But this situation describes a broken-down mechanical device, not a living body. Let's give this a name and call it "macroscopic bias." While blood and lymph might pool under certain circumstances, this represents a *slowing* of circulation, not its cessation. Circulation, chemical transport, and filtration continue constantly, whether we press on an area or not. Bodies are not inherently toxic (with some notable exceptions as a result of disease states), and clients don't need us to flush them in order to be healthy.

Muscles can be released. This one can be tied into myths about lengthening fascia, but it can also stand on its own in this form:

Some muscles stay tight indefinitely, causing all manner of pain and dysfunction, and we can fix that by releasing them.

This idea has appealed to me in the past, because it seems to be true. As you work, you'll feel muscles soften, and occasionally you'll even notice them melt away like hot wax. What is this if not release, and isn't it evidence that we are causing that release? Well, all massage, no matter the modality, seems to promote a reduction in resting muscle tone. In this way we are indeed prompting muscles that would otherwise be tight as a drum to relax, possibly for the first time in months. This is the result of a conversation with the client's nervous system, resulting in the spinal cord inhibiting the feedback loop for the affected stretch receptors, temporarily resulting in lower default motor activity. It feels nice because it is nice.

But those big shifts? Those can be from a more intense interruption of the feedback loop that determines tone (see chapter 3), or from conscious motor activity taking over. Just like you can choose to breathe manually rather than automatically, if you notice that a muscle is staying contracted, you can usually choose to "release" it yourself. Massage can help with this by manually bringing the client's attention to a contracted muscle — they feel your hands distort that tissue, they feel the tightness, and they're able to use that new awareness to relax the muscle.

These are all lovely effects, but I caution you against getting the locus of control wrong. In all these cases, it's the client's own body doing the adjustment to how nerves are firing, with an assist from our hands giving them some new information. It's also temporary. As soon as the client stands up and needs to reorient their body to gravity, they'll tense the muscles that need tension. Any muscle that you "released" on Tuesday will likely be back to its old self on Wednesday. Does that mean that this is all pointless? Of course not, because it's new information for the nervous system to chew on. It might take one repetition or twenty, but eventually, the simple knowledge that it's possible for those tight hip muscles to relax can be enough for the nervous system, either at a conscious level or in the realm of reflexes and feedback loops, to make lasting change.

It has to hurt for it to work. This is a hypothesis common among structural integrators, neuromuscular therapists, and knot proponents alike: Pain is a necessary part of the massage, and we won't get results without it. You've got to breathe through it, or we'll never get that knot out.

But you'll notice something when you dive into the research on massage: Most of it is fairly gentle. Moderate-pressure Swedish and myofascial predominate the successful trials, with some moderate intensity trigger point work also making an appearance. While there are no studies directly comparing painful massage to painless massage, both approaches seem to work in the real world. I've seen this in miniature in my own work: I got results with direct and painful ischemic compression, and I still get results from broad and painless myofascial. My theory is that the body is able to use both stimuli to make changes, and that it doesn't always have a preference for one over the other.

So, my question is this: Even if painful massage works better for some people and some conditions, why jump directly to that when there are other things to try first? Why insist on a type of massage with a more severe side effect profile as your first-line treatment? If you lean toward the painful end of the spectrum, I ask that you try an experiment: Try riding the line of pressure tolerance instead of immediately jumping over it. Find that perfect pressure, or even that "hurts so good" feeling that adds just a touch of nociception to the feel-good sensation. Bring your clients along for this ride: "Joan, I'd like to try some work that's a little less direct, but that should still feel nice and deep. I want to see if it works better for your hip pain, or at least just as well. Is that something you'd be willing to try? Okay great, just let me know if we cross over from deep to painful, because I'll want to back off a bit." Give that a try, ask clients how they feel after, track their progress, and see whether you can default to something a little gentler to start with.

All your problems can be solved by this special system. But only if you come to five week-long classes at two thousand dollars a pop, and do a special internship, and cap it off with advanced training for the *elite* practitioner. In my special system, you'll learn to retrain the nervous system in less than ten seconds, erase pain in one easy session, and fix posture with an extremely specific series of routines. In my special system, you'll learn that the *real* source of pain is the orientation of the feet, or the multifidus muscles, or the first rib! Actually, all pain and dysfunction stems from the big toe, and if we just manipulate it correctly, every other part of the fascial web will fall into its natural alignment.

If any of this sounds familiar, then you've probably been on the hunt for some continuing education lately. There are many mundane offerings meant to shore up your knowledge of prenatal massage or introduce you to Thai massage. And then there are the *systems*. The ones with scientific-sounding names and slick marketing materials and lots of exciting promises about how effective they are. They often have pictures of practitioners applying rather dramatic techniques to clients, usually with their neck or spine in worrisome (yet fascinating!) states of stretch. They seem to promise to let you in on the one true way to work, and the true way to solve pain and dysfunction. You'll find their student evangelists on forums and in comment sections, singing the praises of the system that changed their life, and the lives of so many of their clients.

At this point, I'd like to ask you to take a step back and realize that all massage modalities are made up. All physical therapy regimens and evaluation techniques are made up, even the ones with very scientific sounding names, and many of them are in the process of being left behind by their profession. All surgical approaches were formulated by a person, and then either refined or discarded, with some still being discarded today because they don't seem to work. Freud made up an entire field of psychology — some of it stood the test of time after some refinement, but other parts have been scrapped because they don't seem to have clinical validity.

I'm not saying that "everything is fake and nothing works," I'm saying that we humans are fallible, we're still fumbling around in the dark and trying our best to find out what works, and anyone who claims to have all the answers is not to be taken seriously. Does someone claim to have the answer to low back pain, something that works 100% of the time in one easy session? That, my friends, is a testable hypothesis and a falsifiable claim! Why don't they commission a study and turn the entire field of pain science on its head?

As you can tell, I've got my qualms with these systems with their trademarked names and their incredible claims. The sad part is that I'm sure there are many worthwhile techniques and strategies to be found by taking these courses, but in doing so, students will be bombarded with marketing and persuasion meant to lock you in. And it works! These gurus become very adept at convincing students that they stand at the precipice of true knowledge, just as they convince clients of the same thing. The massage becomes secondary to initiating membership into the inner circle — if you bounce off this process, you miss out on learning the full range of their techniques (often hidden behind many layers of advanced training). If you buy into this new belief system, you change the trajectory of your entire massage career, narrowing your toolset and becoming dogmatic about what "really works."

But, in my experience, the body isn't that simple of a puzzle. There are a hundred ways of working with low back pain, some of them within our scope of practice, and some that will require referring clients out to a physical therapist or acupuncturist. You might have a favorite series of techniques for low back pain that works for a lot of people, but you'll probably find that some people just don't respond to it. The same thing applies in the fields of physical therapy, surgery, and chiropractic. The body is complicated, each client is unique, and what works for one person can't just be copied and pasted onto another person with a 100% success rate.

At the same time, the body can be amazingly adaptive and receptive. Someone with chronic neck pain might find that all they need is good old Swedish to get relief. Or they might just need to add a single daily stretch, or add a few sessions of yoga every week, or change their monitor height. In a lot of ways, the body isn't that picky about the new stimuli it needs to reach a more comfortable equilibrium. So why be dogmatic about which type of massage is the "right way?" Why not keep a broad toolbox, follow your intuition, and see what works?

Lightning round!

Cupping marks are just red blood cells that have followed a pressure gradient, exited the capillaries into surrounding tissues, and become embedded in the dermis and epidermis[34]. This has nothing to do with toxins or stagnant blood, and the different colors likely have to do with small differences in air pressure or local microcirculation.

"Balancing the hips" is a dicey proposition. Using the PSIS landmarks is notoriously unreliable and subject to rater bias[35]. A second massage therapist would likely come to completely different conclusions.

Many postures can be painless, even in the presence of scoliosis, so postural assessment is often a solution in search of a problem. Some postures are associated with pain, as in the case of a client with headaches and head-forward posture. If the client has pain or dysfunction, then pursuing postural change might be worthwhile. But if the client doesn't have posture-related pain? I see no reason to give them a complex about how they stand.

Cannabidiol (CBD) has poor skin permeability, especially if you just dissolve it in some oil[36]. If you use CBD in your practice, avoid homemade preparations, and instead look for products that are designed for absorption. As you ponder these products, realize that we're discussing a pharmacological intervention (albeit one with a benign side effect profile). Whether this is within our scope of practice is currently under debate.

Chances are that you have not found a calcium deposit – most of these are quite small, distributed in the tissue following trauma, and are usually only found via x-ray. If you can palpate something hard and bone-like, you may have located some heterotopic bone (bone that has grown in soft tissue as a response to trauma). In any of the above cases, this isn't something that can or should be "broken

---

34 https://pubmed.ncbi.nlm.nih.gov/22863649/

35 https://www.ncbi.nlm.nih.gov/pmc/articles/PMC4807681/

36 https://www.ncbi.nlm.nih.gov/pmc/articles/PMC7690861/

up" — these are living tissues, and are, by their very nature, much tougher than the surrounding tissue. If you notice a crunchy feel, you're likely feeling connective tissue and/or scar tissue. Work with it as normal, and don't feel the need to try to break it down.

A note on disillusionment

This one's not a myth, but a message for those who have had their notions challenged. I get it. I used to have a strong attachment to the idea that I was changing tissue and restructuring bodies, and learning that this was physically implausible was a blow to my self-image. If I'm not a body mechanic, what am I? The same happened when I learned that the foundation of trigger point theory was much muddier than I had once believed. If trigger points aren't the ultimate answer to musculoskeletal pain, then am I just spinning my wheels?

In short, I had a crisis of faith. I had been a true believer, and then my beliefs got pulled out from under me. I was left feeling adrift and bereft, and it made me question the entire field of massage.

But there were still all those studies where massage had beneficial effects. There were still all those experiences in my own professional life where clients had positive outcomes and amazing experiences. Can that be enough?

You might think, "I wish I had become a physical therapist or orthopedic surgeon. Now those people have rock solid solutions for pain." You might know where I'm going with this, but: Nuh uh. Every conversation we have about the validity of massage and its various modalities? Physical therapists and orthopedists are having those same conversations, often in apocalyptic fashion. Whole swaths of physical therapy best practices are being left behind as we speak, with some people clinging tenaciously to the old ways, and others finding that the new ways are not profoundly more effective. Some surgical interventions are becoming less and less tenable as evidence piles up that they're no more effective than treatment as usual. The surgical gold standards for certain shoulder and knee injuries are in question, and some types of injections are leading to more injury, not less.

So, let's take every profession meant to address musculoskeletal pain and throw them all in a lake, right? Of course not! People find pain relief every day, and often it's not in the first place they look. One physical therapist's approach might exacerbate their pain, while another knocks it right out. They might try surgery for their knee, have a complete relapse of symptoms, and find that massage really does the trick. Or, they might spend a few months trying non-invasive treatments for their carpal tunnel syndrome, eventually give in and get that surgery that their doctor has been after them about, and finally, blissfully, find relief.

So, we're not gods. Neither are PTs or surgeons. Or psychologists, or psychiatrists. Humans are messy, pain is complicated, and massage can be one answer. That also means that we're not the only answer — we're not superior to those other professions, and we don't know better than they do. We're all in this together, and we can be excellent complements to one another.

Remember that massage isn't just about pain, or function, or structure. It's about working with whole people, and supporting them with a unique approach to wellness that you can't find anywhere else in the world. Systematic touch in a nonjudgmental space is a powerful thing for the mind, body, and soul. Can that be enough?

If you're experiencing a crisis of faith as a result of reading this book, or if you came here looking for answers to help with existing disillusionment, know that I've been there, and I got through it. Not because I learned to ignore my misgivings, but because I found all sorts of powerful *stuff* on the other side. There is more to massage than any one technique or any one outcome. Massage is therapy in a very real sense: It is physical therapy, it is psychology, it is meditation, it is yoga and tai chi and maybe even psychedelic therapy. By interfacing with the body through touch, we interface with the mind. By spending time with clients in the shelter we create, we offer a chance to step back from the rest of the world. Even if I weren't able to help with pain, I think that would be enough.

Chapter 11. Massaging Like a Sloth

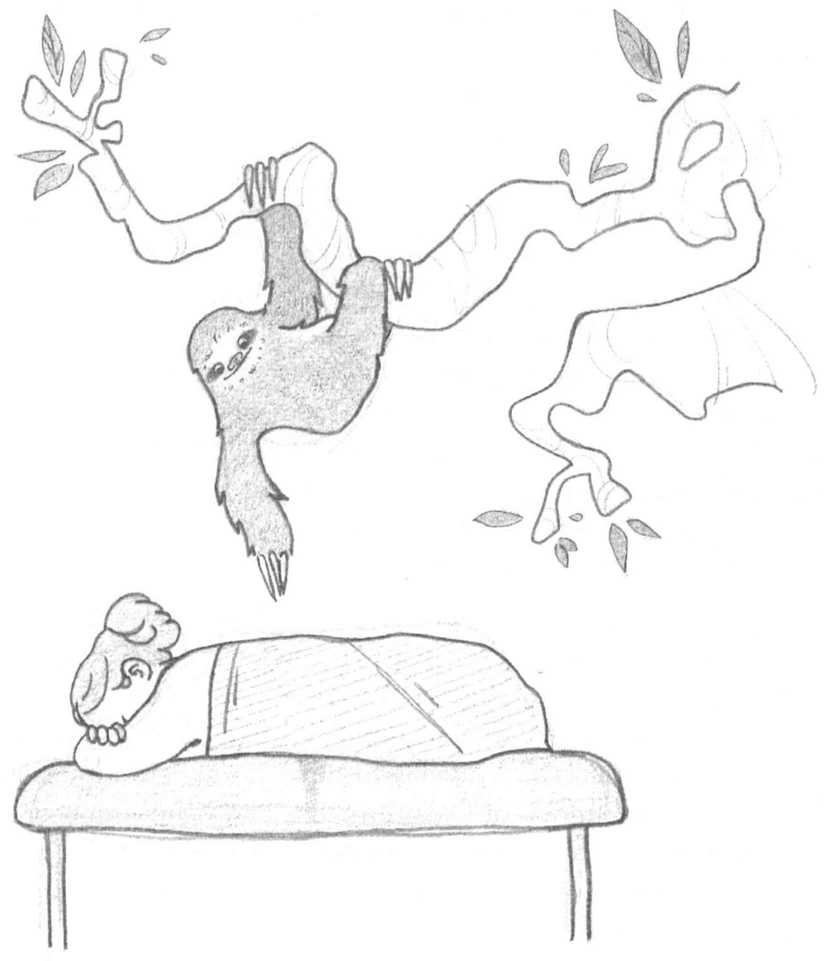

There isn't just one right way to massage, but you're reading my book, so maybe you'd like to know how I go about my work. I've written this chapter as a series of prescriptions, but they should only be followed if you want to be exactly like me. Don't be exactly like me. But *if you wanted to be exactly like me*, here's literally my entire thought process.

Think locally, act globally. Got a client with shoulder pain? Definitely work with that area (don't ignore a primary complaint just because you think it's "coming from somewhere else"), but you should also broaden your perspective and think about everything that might be connected, even tenuously.

What's going on with the neck, any pain there? Any headache? How about down the arm, any numbness or tingling? If the rotator cuff is implicated, don't forget that it's in a tug-of-war with the traps and rhomboids, with the scapula acting as the rope. All of those are in tension with the chest muscles, and the high-tension situation can be exacerbated by a rounded forward posture.

So, keep that shoulder in mind, and then work in lots of other places as well. As you do so, find what seems important to the client, and write it down for future work.

Look for pain connections. I'll talk about frequent patterns that I've found in a moment, but for now: If that client has headaches and upper back pain, what are the odds they're connected? I won't state this as a certainty to the client, but I feel pretty darn certain there's a common factor causing both. I'm looking at you, trapezius and pecs.

Think "lots of stimuli" rather than "the right stimulus." In other words, don't box yourself in by thinking that you need to systematically seek and destroy trigger points, or do 20 minutes of long slow myofascial release in just the right places, or hit exactly the right muscle. Instead, just give their body a lot of new information to chew on.

Here's Ian's Unified Theory of How Massage Works (IUTHMW, pronounced "YUTH-mow"), currently utterly unproven and to be taken with a grain of salt: We provide novel stimuli to the client's central nervous system, and that gives it an opportunity to make changes. Before the massage, the CNS was stuck with days and months of the same stimuli all the time: Office work, Netflix on the couch, sleep. Maybe some exercise on weekends. That's it. During a massage, however, the client's peripheral nervous system reports all sorts of new sensations, including stretch, positioning, and maybe even some nociception.

What will the client's body do with all that new information? Heck if I know! Indeed, according to IUTHMW, it's none of my business. Instead, I just choose to apply a lot of stimuli, from a lot of angles, with the body in interesting positions; I work with areas that are directly connected and long distance; and I see what happens.

A client comes to me with posture concerns related to a protracted head, along with frequent headaches. Do I just do structural integration down their back and up their pecs? Do I just do trigger point work with the anterior neck and the suboccipitals? No! I work in all directions, in all these areas and more. I leave some muscles out because the client finds that work unpleasant. I do a seemingly random mix of modalities. I work with the jaw even though it might be unrelated. Who cares? Not me! I'm leaving it up to the client's nervous system to take this all in, process it however it pleases, and then make changes based on its own internal wisdom. This lets me honor the client's preferences, follow my intuition, do a lot of playing around, and still get good results. Thanks, IUTHMW!

Be lazy. This is really my way of saying "work smart, not hard," and also, "don't overdo it." My favorite way of doing this is to set my table nice and low, prop a thigh against the side, and let gravity take me from point A to point B. Any chance I get to apply a straight arm and lean, I take it.

That's not to say that I never lean way over and use my forearm, it just means that, if I'm going to be doing that, I might as well use *both* my forearms and give the client all my upper body weight, making it a very low-effort situation for me. When I'm not using two active tools, I'll let one hand rest flat on the body, having it act as a "mother hand," a concept I stole from shiatsu. It's comforting, it makes the contact feel bigger and more profound, and it lets me give the client more of my weight. If it sounds like I do a lot of lounging around, you're getting the picture.

I also sit a lot. Not for whole sessions, but if I'm working on the shoulder or hip and I feel like a sit-down, I'll take it. Recognize the unique advantages this gives you: You can rest your forearms on the table. You can approach the body directly from the side. You can rock your body back and forth to generate power or movement, seemingly for free. It's a great angle for manipulating the client's arm, or for applying your forearms just about anywhere.

Finally, I never fatigue myself or my hands. If I can feel myself starting to get tired, I sit. If I know my thumbs are about to get tired, I switch to fists or fingertips. If I've been on a trigger point or doing a myofascial glide for long enough, I switch tools, even if it means making the technique discontinuous. Remember, massage is a forgiving endeavor, and the only thing clients will notice about you switching tools is the enjoyable new sensation.

Let your movements be meaningful. This is another reason to practice putting yourself in the place of your client: It gives you an idea of what you can do with your contact to imbue it with meaning. How can you make the transition from their low back to their upper back feel purposeful and profound instead of strictly utilitarian? In other words, for every moment and every transition, what does your massage *mean*?

I like to think that my massage communicates a message of comfort and safety. When I sink into a muscle, I'm trying to connect with the nervous system rather than just "dig," and the two have a very different feeling to the client. When I squeeze the upper trapezius, I take an extra moment to really experience it, and to let the client do the same. Compare this to how we usually interact with petrissage when we're on autopilot.

Which isn't to say that you can't go on autopilot! That's your cerebellum and motor cortex taking you through your hard-earned motor routines, and it's a great way to reduce the cognitive burden of massage. This lets your hands keep squishing tissue masterfully while you're having those lofty thoughts about meaning, or about curiosity and play.

And once again I'd like to recognize that all this mindful massage stuff can itself be fatiguing. Approach this with a playful and curious attitude as well, rather than thinking of it as a harsh mental regime that needs to be enforced. Do a little here and there, and realize that a mental routine can become automatic, just like a motor routine.

Don't be afraid to slow down. Something that I notice in a lot of massage therapists, especially ones just out of school, is a tendency to race through their techniques. I've got a theory as to why that is: When you slow down, you mentally magnify that time to seem *way* longer than it actually is, and you automatically have worries about what the client is thinking. It's time dilation caused by anxiety. A good solution to the problem of time dilation is to look at an actual clock and time your techniques — ten seconds is a good minimum for a move that irons out the lateral hips, for instance.

As for worries about the client and what they're thinking, realize that knowledge about the contents of someone else's mind in the absence of communication can come from three places: Mind-reading, evidence, and mindfulness. Here's what you'll hear from all three:

1. **Mind-reading**. These are intrusive and automatic thoughts. They're created by worry, and they create worry. A mind-reading thought sounds something like this: "She hates this. This is taking too long for her. He is mad at me. His patience is running out." Mind-reading is usually a form of catastrophizing, and it is usually wrong.
2. **Evidence**. Here you can ask yourself what you know based on past experiences, both regarding yourself and your client. When you receive slower work, does your patience instantly run out? Do you hate every second of a long, luxurious trip down your spinal erectors? Of course not! Does your client have a history of hating your techniques? Nope!
3. **Mindfulness**. Rather than being automatic and intrusive, this is purposeful and empathetic work. Put yourself in your client's place, in their body, on the table. Imagine your hands slowly pausing, or gradually gliding. What does this feel like to you? Maybe, from this new vantage point, you might realize that you could go even slower, or sustain a static compression for longer!

And, of course, you can always just ask. Ask that client, ask other clients, ask trusted friends and colleagues who are on your table. I've learned so much about massage just by finding my voice and speaking up during sessions: "How's this slow work feel? Should I speed up, or is this pace good?"

"I just held that for a good twenty seconds and I'm wondering about that experience for you. Was that too long, or do you wish it had gone on longer? It was perfect and I totally nailed it? Okay, great!"

I think you'll find that your clients like slow work just as much as you do, and that slowing down can open the door to some really profound and powerful ways of interacting with the body. Slowness says, "let's take time to really consider this part of the body. What's going on here, and how is it changing?" It creates an environment where the "melt" of myofascial release can happen, or the deactivation of neuromuscular therapy. While I disagree with some of the theory underlying these modalities, these shifts that the body goes through are very real nervous system phenomena, and they only tend to happen when you give them time to. Another stimulus to play with!

Be a force of nature. Let gravity do the work during the massage, and let it rock the client's body. I talked about this in the context of being lazy above, but I also want you to conceptualize it as a way of changing the client's experience on the table. Consider these two ways of working:

In the first version of this stroke, you use your loose fist to travel down the client's erector spinae muscles. You're focused on stripping those muscles out specifically, so your intention is only an inch deep. Your table is at waist height, bringing the surface of the client's body up to your belly button. This forces the movement to come from the extension of your arm, and maybe some rotation at your hips. You repeat this move several times with alternating fists, bearing down using your pecs and triceps so that the pressure is deep enough to meet your client's preference.

In the second version of this stroke, mentally lower the table by about six to twelve inches, and mentally remove about 75% of the oil or lotion on the client's body. Their back is now situated at or below your waist, and any technique will have to be a slow glide. You apply a fist an inch to the side of your client's spine, and then you straighten your arm and your posture. From there, you lean forward, toward the client's feet, allowing your fist to slowly travel inferiorly. As your fist glides, your intention is to pour your body weight deep into your client, allowing it to change the orientation of their ribs, and their spine, and eventually their pelvis. The erector spinae muscles still get some nice stripping, but it's in the context of a technique that *feels* much deeper, even if the physical pressure ends up being similar.

Think about the different ways that these strokes will be perceived by the client on the table. The first technique, the one that comes from the strength of the arm and the shoulder, will feel nice! It might also feel a little shaky and inconsistent, with the pressure tapering off as you lose leverage. The second technique, driven by the movement of your whole body and translated through a straight arm, will be anything but shaky — it will feel consistently strong and confident. As the fist makes its way from the thoracic region to hips, changing shape to conform to the client's body as it does so, the client will feel their body change shape as well. Their ribs will compress, their vertebrae will experience some extension and rotation, and the entire spine will be drawn into light traction as the fist sinks into the lower back and upper gluteal region.

Surface-level stripping is a fine technique, and a good tool to have in your toolbox, but by and large, I want my massage to be remembered as a force of nature. I want it to feel like a landslide, or a crashing wave. Be bold with your massage, and use your whole body as you work.

If any of this seems intimidating, the answer is, once again, communication! Let your client (or friend, or colleague) know that you're going to be experimenting with throwing your weight around, and have them give you feedback on what feels good, and what feels like too much. Mentally put yourself in the place of your client and try to anticipate where it will feel nice to have the full weight of your body sink in, and where it can be good to lean back a bit and lower the pressure. This is a big paradigm shift, so ease into it, and expect some false starts.

Oh, and if you'd like to get a crash course on using your body weight fearlessly, take a Thai massage workshop. Once you've spent a weekend crawling on and around a few fellow practitioners (and hearing how great it feels), you'll get a new sense of how bold you're allowed to be in your movements.

Make every contact a question. It's possible to make every contact with the body feel like you're laying claim, like an explorer planting a flag on unexplored country. I think this tends to happen when massage therapists get really interested in *skipping to the good stuff* rather than worrying about all the little peripheral elements that make massage relaxing and comforting. If you're going to work out all those knots, there's no time for warming up the tissue for more than ten seconds, and I certainly can't be bothered to float around like I'm doing tai chi!

But, of course, you can spare the time, and it's time well spent. It's a matter of meaning: A quick contact will mean something to the client, and it will be very different from the message conveyed by something more gradual. You can choose to be mindful every time your hands make contact with the body, descending at a measured pace and conforming to the body's unique shape. This is something that the teachers at my alma mater, the Florida School of Massage, call the *airplane landing*. As you do this, you can silently ask some questions: "What is it that I'm feeling under my hands?" and "May I?"

These gradual contacts can be an extension of your efforts to reduce the power differential. By taking your time and acknowledging their body's unique shape, you're giving them time to consider your touch, and time to consider their own body. It can prompt them to ask the question, "what is this part of my body like? Is this touch okay?" And, because you're moving at a measured and predictable pace, they have the time to say, "actually, could we skip that part today?" And you have the time to track their breathing, and their body, and see whether a contact is causing them to tense up. It can all be an extension of the groundwork of communication that you've been laying, and it can reinforce the concept of seeking robust consent.

Oh, and these slow landings and takeoffs feel nice! Mindful and meaningful touch can be effortful at first, but like all other mindfulness exercise, you'll find they become easier and more accessible over time.

How the body fits together

There have been a number of researchers, physical therapists, and massage therapists who have gone into great detail explaining their concept of how the body relates to itself. Travell and Simons were very definite about where trigger points live and the regions that they refer to, almost making it seem like these are all part of self-evident natural law and consistent from person to person (despite trigger points proving elusive and of debatable relevance in subsequent research). There have been those who describe myofascial meridians with supreme surety, and others who trumpet the all-important role of tensegrity. For others, cerebrospinal fluid and its circulation are the ultimate explanation of how the body relates to itself, and the answer to all manner of dysfunction.

Well, if everyone else can have their own pet theory about how the body works, then so can I. I won't give my system a name, but please pretend that it's all very official and scientific, and that none of it whatsoever is based on flawed observations, personal biases, or false patterns that my brain constructed from incomplete information. No, this was all handed to me by the gods of massage, whole and incontrovertible! Let's start from the top.

Headaches are about the face, neck, and shoulders. When a client reports frequent headaches, make sure to ask them to point out where they feel pain. If it's in the temples, ask, "any pain or dysfunction in your jaw?" You'll often find that people forget about jaw pain and regard it as their lot in life, so reminding them of this can open a fruitful new avenue of approach. Whether they have jaw pain or not, work with their masseter, temporalis, and sternocleidomastoid. You might even find trigger points in the SCM that refer directly into the temples. If so, give that section of SCM enough of a squeeze to activate that referral, ask your client to take some easy, deep breaths, and wait for the referral to fade. No, you haven't erased a trigger point, but you have demonstrated to the nervous system that there is a connection, and that it can be less reactive.

If they point to their forehead, ask about the base of their skull, and vice versa. These seem to have a reciprocal referral relationship, and both seem to be based on superior trapezius yanking on the occipital region. Work with the occiput, the entire trapezius (yes, even lower traps), the pecs, and the rotator cuff. All of these can be engaged in a tug-of-war that leaves trapezius chronically tight and irritated. If you find a trigger point in the occipital region, even a really juicy one, please err on the side of doing too little. Limit the intensity and duration of your contact, and see how they respond. In my experience, it's easy to overdo it with direct occipital work, and a little goes a long way.

Oh, and with any headache, don't forget about face and scalp massage. Think long, slow drags.

Neck pain is about front vs. back, and about the shoulders. If a client has posterior neck pain, I'm interested in the forces pulling the neck and shoulders forward. What are those posterior muscles fighting against? SCM, scalenes, and pecs loom large in my mind. I'll work with the posterior neck as well, with long slow strips up the paraspinals, and long cranial cradles. For self-care, short duration "chin tucks" (neck retractions that give you a double chin) can help the body get a better sense of how to defuse that anterior tension. As with all exercises, only suggest them if it's within your personal expertise and your scope of practice.

For "neck cricks," we're usually dealing with spasm and sensitivity of the levator scapulae. Have your client turn their head to the restricted side, then point directly to where they feel that sensation of pain and restriction. I'm betting they'll point to the transverse process of a cervical vertebra, which is a pretty clear indication that levator is acting up. Work with levator while keeping them in a comfortable range of motion, and consider working with upper traps, SCM, and the pecs as well, just to keep things broad. Repeat the head turning test, have them point to their pain (if it moved, or if their range of motion is improved, you're on the right track), then give them one more repetition of the direct levator work.

I like long slow compression for this, pinning the superior angle of the scapula with one hand while the other contacts the lateral neck.

Some clients will have anterior neck stuff, which might include changes in how they swallow, how they talk, or how they sing. Their first resource here will be their physician, who will hopefully refer them to a speech-language pathologist. You can also encourage them to seek a referral to a physical therapist or occupational therapist who specializes in the neck and throat. We can offer a gentle adjunct to the treatment they're receiving from their medical team by adding some long, slow myofascial drags to the anterior and lateral neck each session. Stay well within your client's comfort zone, consider working unilaterally if it feels "chokey," and don't forget SCM, pecs, and jaw work. Creating traction down the sternum while they gently nod or do neck retractions can be an excellent fascial stretch for the entire anterior neck.

Shoulder pain is about the rotator cuff, pecs, traps, and rhomboids. If your client reports shoulder pain, start by having them point it out. Most people will point directly to the front of their glenohumeral joint, which is right around the insertion site of subscapularis. Should we just attack subscap and call it a day? No! My theory here is that all the rotator cuff muscles have tightened up to brace the shoulder (maybe we're dealing with a dental hygienist who spends all day doing excruciatingly fine shoulder movements, or even a desk worker doing the same thing), and poor subscap is just clinging on for dear life, trying to deal with this high-tension environment. The more that we can have a conversation with all four rotator cuff muscles, and with the pecs pulling forward, and with the traps and rhomboids pulling back, the happier subscapularis will be. Of course, some direct work with subscap can be lovely — sandwich the scapula, with your thumb pads pressing deep into the axilla, and flat fingers cupping the posterior scap, and you'll be on it. This can be very gentle, and should be done with robust informed consent.

What about pain deep in the joint, or pain around back? I hate to break it to you, but my approach will be much the same. We're still dealing with a tug-of-war dynamic that can use an overall reduction in tension, and I'd rather give the area a lot of input and let it decide how to find a new normal. If any of this shoulder stuff is persistent or is causing difficulty with activities of daily living, please encourage your client to see their doctor for evaluation.

And I'd be remiss if I didn't talk about frozen shoulder. Some people gradually or rapidly lose the ability to bring their shoulder into abduction or external rotation, with the sensation becoming rather scary and feeling like structural damage (even when no damage can be found). This seems to be from a neurological habit of dysfunctional spasm — if you get a client with frozen shoulder on your table, this makes your job pretty simple. Give their nervous system evidence, week after week, that there is no crisis. Cradle their arm, gently wrap their shoulder in warm and confident hands, and do some long, slow myofascial drags of the entire shoulder region. Then, compress that head of the humerus toward the glenoid fossa and take their arm through a tiny range of motion. See, nervous system? No damage here. Just good vibes. Over time, as you identify movements and actions that feel safe for your client, you can increase that range of motion, and even have them engage in some active movements as you work. Let safety and comfort guide you, and you'll do well.

Hand and wrist pain are about the forearm and shoulder. Give me an achy hand or a tender wrist, and my first thought is about the wrist flexors and extensors and how they're being used. Work with the muscular portions all the way to their origin at the epicondyles rather than focusing just on the tendons in the wrist and hand. Apply some nice slow myofascial strokes proximally as the client engages in some gentle movements.

And then, expand your view broadly, and work all the way up to the shoulder and beyond. Think about what muscles and structures might be impinging the brachial plexus, and work beyond their origins and insertions. Spend time with the pecs, rotator cuff (these can be surprisingly relevant, sometimes referring pain directly to the site in question), traps, and scalenes. Work with the arm and shoulder in different positions rather than leaving it on the table. Nothing makes the chest feel open like pec work while the shoulder is flexed up and away from the ribs.

If your client has numbness or tingling in their fingers, let that be your guide. If they feel it in their thumb, index finger, and middle finger (digits 1-3), or in the region of the anterior wrist, then we're dealing with impingement of the median nerve. This could be at the carpal tunnel, but it might be having an interaction with the wrist flexors. Iron those out, along with the extensors for good measure, then continue up to work with the elbow flexors and extensors. Don't attack the nerve directly (you can easily interact with nervous and vascular tissue on the medial side of the humerus, so make sure to stay on muscle), but iron out the biceps and brachialis in broad slow strips, including some slow extension of the elbow.

If your client has numbness in digits 4 and 5, then we're dealing with some problem with the ulnar nerve. This might also be felt in the ulnar side of the palm, including the area of the pisiform bone. Working with the wrist flexors and extensors is wise here, but I often find that this has something to do with the interplay of the elbow flexors and extensors, and ironing out the triceps can help. Be mindful of the area posterior to the medial epicondyle where the ulnar nerve is superficial and easily pinned against bone (the area colloquially known as the "funny bone") — indeed, ask the client if they find themselves resting that area on the armrests of their desk chair. If so, they need to use lower arm rests, or to use a chair without armrests while their arm recovers. 8 hours of pressure per day can be enough to upset any nerve.

In both of the cases above, make sure to continue your work up to the shoulder and beyond, just in case the impingement is actually higher up in the brachial plexus, before the individual nerves branch off. For all hand, wrist, and forearm symptoms, I like to recommend gentle wrist stretches, as well as stretching of the pecs. A rounded forward shoulder with tight pecs can easily start clamping down on nerves and vasculature as they pass.

Upper back pain is about a tug-of-war. If a client tells me that their upper back is killing them, then mashing on that upper back isn't my primary focus (though I will do some feel-good work there). Instead, I'm thinking of all the structures that are pulling the shoulders into protraction, as well as the forces pulling the head forward. Imagine how the rhomboids and trapezius must feel in such a situation, spending 16 hours a day at maximum stretch while resisting gravity with all their might. You'd be angry too!

Once I've had a conversation with these clients about broadening our scope, I'll spend plenty of time with the pecs, SCMs, and rotator cuff. The rotator cuff muscles might not seem like an obvious target, but think about what they do when they all fire at once: They glue the scapula out laterally, keeping it tight to the upper humerus. Convincing the rotator cuff group to chill out can be a big relief to the upper back. I always recommend pec stretches to people with upper back pain, and chin tucks would be a good bet as well.

Also, if you're seeing a pattern here, you've caught on to one of my theories about upper body pain: That most of it is about the tug-of-war between front and back, and that if we could get the anterior muscles to chill out and allow the body to comfortably stand erect, those posterior muscles would be happier. We can help with this using massage and self-care recommendations, but part of this will be down to convincing the clients to take more frequent breaks at work, and to be more active in ways that encourage them to stand up tall (e.g., yoga, running, weight training... pretty much any active endeavor). You don't need to be dogmatic about this, or make it a condition for continuing to work, or anything like that. Just the occasional mention is usually enough.

Low back pain is about the hips. *Sometimes* it's clearly centered on the QL region, but in most cases, when I have someone point to their "low back pain," they'll point directly to their SI joint. I'll still make plenty of contact with the actual lumbar region as a way of working broadly, but I'm much more interested in every muscle that attaches near that SI region, as well as their antagonists.

When someone comes to me with low back or hip pain, I make sure to ask these questions: "Any pain or tingling down the leg?" "Any pain along the front of your hip or groin?" If they've got symptoms that travel down the leg, make sure to note where and when they feel them, then track these symptoms over time. For these clients (and all clients with low back and hip pain) I'll work with the posterior and lateral hip muscles, steamrolling them and compressing them while sometimes drawing the leg into internal rotation. You can do plenty of good work with the gluteus medius/minimus while the client is prone and supine, rocking the leg as you sink in with a fist or group of fingertips (these lateral muscles might not seem directly related, but I've encountered many sensitive gluteus medius muscles in people with posterior pain).

For clients with pain along the anterior pelvis, this is usually centered on the inguinal ligament. I'll explain that "you've got a ligament here that acts as a sling for the hip flexors, which lie deep in your abdomen and pelvis, and which attach to the inner thigh here. These muscles get activated powerfully every time you run or do a sit-up, and they're kept in a shortened position whenever you sit. I'd like to work with those muscles and get them to calm down a bit, which should be useful for this pain up front, and the pain in your glutes around back. Is that something you'd like to try?" Upon getting this general consent, I'll make sure to explain the process of working with iliacus and psoas before I do so, getting specific informed consent.

Basically, when you've got a low back pain client with symptoms centered on their pelvis, do your best to educate them about their various hip flexors and extensors, and then work with those muscles in a lot of interesting positions. If a client is prone to back spasm, or if they tend to get up from a massage table with a stiff back, try making some changes to their positioning: A pillow under the lower abdomen will keep them from having a hyperlordotic lumbar region while prone, and a large bolster under the knees while supine will do the same. If neither of these does the trick, then use more side-lying positioning. In other words, if you're able to keep these clients in something closer to a fetal position during their massage, their hypersensitive low back will thank you for it.

I like to send these clients home with a gentle kneeling lunge stretch. Place a pillow on the floor, have them kneel on it while placing a hand on a nearby wall or piece of furniture for support, then have them shift their body weight forward. As they do so, they'll need to tip their pelvis posteriorly, which is easiest to describe like this: "As you lunge forward, think of tucking your tailbone. Do you feel that stretch along the front of your hip?" I have them repeat slowly, coming into and out of the stretch about as fast as they breathe, for about 5 repetitions, then switch. My reasoning is this: There's a tug-of-war happening between the front and back of the pelvis, and because of daily sitting for 10+ hours, the flexors are used to being short. By implementing a daily lunge stretch regimen, we can get one side of that battle to lay down their arms, potentially giving everything on the posterior side a bit of a break.

Just know that low back pain is a tough nut to crack, especially when there's spasm involved (their back "goes out."). Think of massage as a gradual desensitization process over the course of many sessions, convincing those hip extensors and external rotators to loosen their death grip on the posterior pelvis and their compression of the sciatic nerve. Working with the lateral and anterior hip muscles can help. Be patient with this, find out what provokes spasm and avoid it, and make changes to positioning as needed. Encourage these clients to try stretching and other activities, and recommend physical therapy to clients who have substantial difficulty or pain.

Knee pain is... complicated. When you have a client with knee pain, ask where they feel it. If it's on the medial side of the patella, I'm thinking of vastus medialis needing some work. If it's on the outer side, then I suspect vastus lateralis and the IT band. If it's centered directly on the patella, feels like it's under the patella, or is just distal to the patella (i.e., runner's knee), then I'll work broadly with the quads and IT band tensors. If the pain feels deep in the leg joint rather than related to the patella, or even on the posterior knee, then I start to suspect gastrocnemius and the hamstrings. In that case I'll work with the calf in lots of interesting positions along with the thigh.

A note on working with the IT band: No amount of stripping or stretching will affect the length of the IT band itself. A much more workable solution is to target the muscles that put tension on that band, namely tensor fasciae latae (TFL) and gluteus maximus. Steamroll out the glutes, compress them while rolling the femur into internal rotation, and then target TFL. This is easiest to do by finding the anterior superior iliac spine (ASIS), coming just inferior, and feeling for a little muscle that jumps up when the client internally rotates their hip. From there you can do some compressions with your fist or fingertips while the client does some gentle rocking of the leg back and forth.

Can't remember what to do with a particular presentation of knee pain? Then just do what I usually do and work broadly. Work with the medial and lateral thigh, hit the gastrocs, and work with the hips. It takes some extra time, but this broad focus can be beneficial to all sorts of clients with knee pain, whether it be from osteoarthritis or running.

Foot pain is about the calf. At least, it's the first place my mind goes. When someone comes to me with achy feet, or the characteristic walking-on-broken-glass feeling near the heel that typifies plantar fasciitis, I usually find calves that are tight as a drum and usually quite strong. If I ask them to plantarflex they can point their foot straight down, but their dorsiflexion is usually quite limited. If this is all true, then my plan is clear: Lots of work with the posterior low leg, and an easy stretching regimen as self-care.

The work looks like this: I use paired fists to do long, slow ironing out of the calf, starting from the Achilles tendon and travelling all the way to the popliteal region (the posterior knee), at which point I lighten up and make sure my pressure is directed toward the head rather than down toward the table. I do some repetitions, often recruiting them to bring their ankle into subtle dorsiflexion repeatedly as I do so. If the table is in their way, put a larger bolster under their ankle, or hang their foot off the edge of the table (which can be uncomfortable for some people's knees, so be aware). From here you can pluck up the ankle and work with the calf while you pump their foot into dorsiflexion, followed by some ironing out of the anterior and lateral low leg.

For self-care, I have them stand in a lunge position with one hand on a wall for support. I demonstrate that their foot should be straight forward rather than allowed to point out to the side (that's cheating), then have them shift their weight forward while their rear foot remains flat on the floor. If they feel a gentle stretch in their posterior low leg, then they're doing it right. I have them pulse into and out of the stretch five times, as quickly as they breathe, and then have them switch sides. Suggest that they do this several times throughout their day, perhaps whenever they get up to go to the bathroom at work.

My Million Dollar Moves

That heading might be a little overdramatic. Let's just call this section "how I differentiate myself and wow my clients." These are the techniques and strategies I use that seem somewhat rare in the massage world, and that are both effective and enjoyable for the recipient. I invite you to take them and make them your own. If you'd like to see these in action, check out the resources page at massagesloth.com/booksupplement where I have links to each of these on my YouTube channel. Did I mention that I see no point in hoarding my knowledge and that I find it useful (and fun!) to just give it away? I invite you to take that strategy too.

Scooping the scapula. This one is about mobilizing the scapula, even if you can't get under it or even define all its borders on a particular body. Use the curved fingers of one hand to cradle the superior angle of the scapula and use the other hand to pinch the inferior angle. From there you can wiggle the entire scap, you can bring it into protraction and retraction, you can move it superiorly and inferiorly. Depending on the client's muscle tone and overlying adipose tissue, you might be able to pinch all the way under the scapula, lifting it from the underlying ribs. From here you can lean back, drawing the shoulder blade up and away, decompressing all the underlying bursae and giving them a reason to hydrate.

The pec/neck fascial stretch. Sit at one corner of the table near the head. Place an open palm on the client's upper chest, and a loose fist on their upper traps. Let your chest hand press laterally while the fist travels up the neck. There seems to be a fascial connection between these two areas, and bringing them into stretch in this way can help the client stand up with a new sense of freedom in how they hold their head. It also just feels amazing. Yes, this is the one that I call the "Harvey Maneuver." It started as a joke, I swear.

Exploring the pecs. While we're in the area, we might as well place the client's hand over our arm and then walk our thumbs under pec major. From here you can simply make a pec sandwich, rocking your own body to take the client's shoulder through some subtle rotation. Explore all the way up to the insertion at the upper humerus — the pec major tendon enjoys some direct attention.

Glutes up, down, and sideways. The glutes and other hip muscles are the connection between the upper and lower body. They're the unsung heroes of standing, walking, and sitting, and they typically spend their lives without much human contact. When you work with them, consider approaching them from different directions: From the top down as you work with the back, from the bottom up as you work with the legs, and with fascial traction away from the SI joint toward the greater trochanter. Any client who has never received thorough glute work before will instantly feel the significance and profoundness of this work.

Specific neck work. Here I'm talking about using your fingers to directly compress the levator scapulae while restraining its attachment to the superior angle of the scapula. Grasping sternocleidomastoid gently, and waiting. Defining the upper and lower border of the clavicle, bowling over the inferior scalenes as you do so. Following upper trapezius superiorly as it becomes thin and ribbon-like. Really tell the story of these muscles as you work with them.

The rib zamboni. This is any move that makes a big, broad contact with the thoracic region and scoops it superiorly or toward the spine. Having someone take a full minute or two to press your rib fascia toward your head can make it seem extra easy to take a breath once you stand up.

Compressing the ischium. A long stroke up the hamstring that ends with sustained upward compression of the ischial tuberosity can feel like it's decompressing your low back. A sustained downward compression starting from the upper ilium can do the same thing. It is a mystery.

Upturned fingers. Have a seat and place both hands on the massage table, palm up. Curl your fingers slightly. You now have a crowbar that you can walk underneath a supine client's back and use to press upwards into their thoracic ribs, infraspinatus, erector spinae, and even QL, all just by keeping that same shape and dropping your elbows toward the floor. By making the shape with your hands and then moving your arms, this can be almost effortless for your wrist and finger flexors, and the client's weight does all the work.

The foot grasp-and-lean. Use both hands to grasp the foot of a supine client, with your fingertips sinking into the plantar surface. Now, just lean back and glide distally. A much easier way of stripping the intrinsic foot muscles than using your thumbs, and it feels fantastic.

The two-fisted steamroller. Place two soft fists on the client's lumbar region, palms toward you. Sink your knuckles into the spinal erectors as you drag toward yourself, taking the thoracolumbar fascia for a ride laterally. A long, slow, sustained drag, with your bodyweight over your client, feels great for the low back, and it addresses the QL in an indirect way rather than the usual pinpoint pressure. If your contact is broad and follows your client's unique shape, there will be no pressure on the floating ribs.

The cranial cradle. Use both hands to strip up either side of the cervical spine of a supine client, ending near the occiput. Now, curl your fingers, allowing the client's skull to rest in your upturned claw hands. By having their occipital region resting on eight fingertips, this creates a "bed of nails" effect where the small supports don't feel sharp because there are so many of them. It also feels like floating. Hold this for at least 30 seconds, then allow your fingers to melt before you slowly sneak out the sides.

Interlude: Things You Always Wanted to Know about Massage But Were Too Afraid to Ask

What do I do if a client has a lot of body hair? Nothing much! Hair follicles are usually fairly insensitive. Not as in rude, but as in "doesn't feel much," especially when good pressure is applied. Can you imagine being aware of your back hair every time you sit down or put on a shirt? Doesn't happen, the nervous system just filters those inputs out. The same goes for most leg hair (posterior and medial thigh follicles can be a little sensitive, however), arm hair, and chest hair.

On a practical level you might find that it changes your ability to flow along the skin. Your first impulse might be to add lots of oil or lotion, but only do that if that's your usual default. If you prefer little or no lotion, try that on your hairy clients, and ask about their experience. "Does this feel like your hair is getting pulled at all? Okay great, just keep me updated." You might even find that you need *less* oil than usual, with the hair buoying your technique along.

My one caveat: Be careful with highly vigorous work on hairy skin, especially making lots of small circles. I've had to alter my sports massage to be slower and broader on some clients when the frequent changes in direction became irritating to their follicles. Usually not a problem, but something to keep in mind for faster work.

How do I work with clients with lots of body fat? I frequently get these questions on videos where I'm demonstrating work with a specific muscle: If I can't see the muscle on a particular client, how do I work with it? How can I reach the muscle if there's a layer of fat on top? The good news is that there's very little you need to change. Subcutaneous fat does distribute force out radially, but the effect is fairly minimal, and you should still be able to give their muscles work that feels intense and direct through inches of adipose tissue. If you can't see the muscle, you should still be able to isolate it by palpating it during active engagement, or approximating its position using landmarks.

The same goes for myofascial release and structural integration: There's not much you need to change. Realize that the superficial fascia (the subcutaneous region, including the fat) is continuous with the deep fascia; there is no point at which it is "glued on," the collagenous web is all one piece! By moving the skin and underlying fat, we're interfacing directly with the deepest parts of the body, and that remains the same no matter the volume of embedded adipose tissue. Place the skin over the scapula in myofascial traction, and it will be felt in the rotator cuff.

My main concern with larger clients is their comfort on the table. Clients with larger breasts might appreciate a higher face cradle and rolled up towels under their shoulders (or a specialized cut-out bolster). Clients with lots of muscle or body fat might find that their arms tend to spill over the edges of the table; this can be a good time to have width extenders that you can strap to the table prior to the session. If this happens unexpectedly during a session, you can have them tuck their hands under their upper hip region on each side while prone, which keeps their arms from migrating outward. While supine, they might be more comfortable in a semi-reclined position, or with a small pillow under their head. As always, your client is your best resource.

What if a client has cancer, or a chronic illness, or a recent surgery? I know that's a whole lot to pack into one question, but there are some fairly simple rules to follow here. First and foremost, the best antidote to fear is knowledge. Grab yourself a copy of *A Massage Therapist's Guide to Pathology: Critical Thinking and Practical Application* by Ruth Werner and spend a little time every day making your way through it. Afterwards you'll have a better grip on how to think about just about any disease state you might encounter, and you'll know what questions to ask clients who present with these conditions. You can keep this text on your bookshelf and refer to it any time anything new pops up on an intake form, or even in the middle of a client interview if you'd like to double check your memory. You would also be well served by taking some continuing education classes directly related to cancer care, many of which can be found online. I recommend Tracy Walton's workshops for a detailed and compassionate treatment of the topic.

Second, if a client has been put on activity restrictions by their doctor or surgeon, let those point you in the right direction. For example, if a client is on bedrest, either postpone the massage until they're in a less vulnerable state, or stick with non-contact and minimal-contact modalities such as Reiki or Polarity. If a client can go on a walk, they can probably tolerate light Swedish or other non-invasive modalities that are unlikely to cause inflammation or circulatory trauma. Someone who can go on a jog can probably receive a fairly vigorous massage, and a client who can jump back into full-tilt CrossFit can get any type of massage they please.

Third, respect inflammation and circulatory vulnerability. Avoid surgical sites and areas distal to them until inflammation subsides, unless you have specific training for working with post-surgical areas, such as manual lymphatic drainage. If a client has had lymph nodes removed, limit the duration and intensity of your massage in a related limb until you determine how prone that area is to lymphedema. If a client has a history of blood clots or is otherwise susceptible to them, avoid provoking tissue damage in the limbs, and be scrupulous about your strokes moving from distal to proximal.

Finally, be aware that recovery is rarely a straight line. This goes for recovery from surgery, physical therapy for an injury, and improvements in the symptoms of a chronic illness. If you're working with a client with post-concussion syndrome and things are going great — their headaches are less frequent, their fatigue and brain fog are improving, and their mood is lifting — it can be disheartening, and even scary, when things take a turn for the worse. Did all your hard work go down the drain? Are you both back to square one? No, because relapse is part of recovery. If you were to look at a chart of anyone's recovery from an illness or injury, you'd see a graph with gradual improvements, frustrating plateaus, and sudden precipitous drops representing re-injuries and flare-ups of old symptoms. But if you were to zoom way out, you'd see that the general trend was upward, and that those setbacks were just part of the process all along. That's something that you can keep in mind as you work, and it's an important message that you can pass along to clients who might be discouraged.

Shouldn't I ask for a doctor's note? This is another meme that floats around massage communities that seems to have little basis in best practice or the prevention of medical errors. It tends to sound like this: If someone has a condition that seems scary or unusual, you should "cover your bases" or "reduce your liability" by asking them to get written permission from their doctor prior to receiving massage.

Let's imagine the best-case scenario here: The client makes an appointment with their orthopedist, oncologist, or general practitioner, explains that their massage therapist has requested permission to do work, and the doctor has the front desk print out a page that says, "this patient has been cleared for massage." You put this note in your client's file and proceed, feeling more secure in having done your due diligence.

In truth, this delay in care has accomplished very little. At no point in this process have you sidestepped your duty to prevent medical errors, and you probably haven't reduced your liability. If a client is injured by massage, a doctor's note is unlikely to change how much your liability insurance pays out or whether you're sanctioned by your certifying body — it is always incumbent on you as the massage therapist to follow best practices for all clients, including those with medical vulnerabilities. A note shouldn't affect your decision-making process regarding how to proceed, because you are the expert on massage in this client's healthcare team.

A note is also unlikely to be informative. Doctors tend not to know much about massage (they usually imagine a generic Swedish routine), and we shouldn't assume otherwise unless we've done the work to inform them, or to seek out a referral network that values and understands bodywork as healthcare. An exception to all the above is if you need more information about the client's condition before you proceed. If the client is unsure about whether their last venous ultrasound found clots, you might choose not to work with that limb until they've phoned their doctor and asked for clarification. If you've got specialized training in a field of pathology, you might even ask your client to get you copies of certain scans or test results which might guide your treatment plan.

You can also feel free to have your client ask about massage without making it a prerequisite for their next session. That might sound something like this: "I'm glad your surgery went well! At your next physical therapy appointment, would you ask about a timeline for massage? I want to follow their lead here, and they'll have useful insight into how your recovery is going." I've made a number of friends among local physical therapists by coordinating with them through clients, and by advocating for PT when a client has new or unresolved pain. Physical and occupational therapists will also be likely to have a good grasp on manual therapy and its applications.

Before I leave this topic, I'd like to mention the worst-case scenario when you require a doctor's note prior to working on a client: The client sees this as too high a hurdle, or they see it as a rejection, and they simply never come back. This is a way that already stigmatized people (e.g., those living with HIV/AIDS, people with cancer, elders) can be further stigmatized, and effectively be denied care that could have been a boon, or even a turning point in their lives. Yes, follow your gut and use your best clinical judgment, but keep in mind that healthcare delayed can easily become healthcare denied.

Do I need to stop playing the guitar/climbing/doing martial arts? Are my hands going to explode? Please, I beg you, do not start narrowing your activities to try to be the optimal massage therapist. First of all, cross-training is important for your health and long-term viability in this field. Giving your body lots of different stimuli through a variety of postures, fine movements, and muscle pattern activations will send the signal that you require flexibility and versatility rather than strict adaptation to a single type of activity. The same goes for your brain: Lots of different enjoyable (and even difficult-but-surmountable) stimuli will be a better engine for growth and resilience than a single repetitive task.

Secondly, your hobbies are more important than your work. Your work can be your calling, yes, but hobbies are how you express your multidimensionality. They're how you nurture your inner artist and adventurer, and how you give voice to your subconscious mind. "Ian, we're talking about crocheting here." Yeah, we're talking about crocheting! When your fingers are flying through a pattern and you've reached that pleasant state of flow where your hands feel self-motivated and you're in touch with your power as a creator, that's a treasure worth protecting. When you're sweating through your uniform and ready to throw in the towel, and then suddenly the kata just clicks? When your effort becomes effortless, that's when the world rises to meet you.

So, keep your hobbies, *but...* if you notice that an activity seems to be conspiring with massage to cause hand pain or back pain, that is a time to make a change. I recommend making that change in the massage room — find ways to take the load off that body part. Use more fists and forearms, and sit more often. Also, consider adding *more* activity! Some strength training for your hands and hips (and everything else) could allow you to do your work and your hobbies with ease. What used to be fatiguing will now be well within your capability, and you'll still get to go home and put in that hour of guitar practice.

I noticed a lump or unusual mole on my client. Should I tell them about it? The most important thing to note here is that most people are already aware of their moles, lumps, and bumps. In fact, you can phrase it with that in mind: "Jim, I notice a lump here next to your spine. Is that something you're aware of?" The answer is almost always yes, and they'll fill you in on what it is and whether it's painful. These under-skin lumps are usually lipomas, which are benign fatty tumors that don't feel like much of anything to the client.

For moles that might need further evaluation (larger than a dime, irregular borders, uneven appearance, mottled coloration), you can use a similar phrasing following the session. "Jim, I noticed a mole on your back that looked slightly irregular to me. Is that something you're aware of?" If they say no, just say, "okay, just do me a favor and mention that to your doctor next time you see them." Delivering this with brisk professionalism will send the message that this is all normal and routine, and that they don't need to worry.

Indeed, they don't need to worry! Most lumps, especially stable and soft ones, are benign. Most moles are benign. Even in the case of precancerous or cancerous lesions, most types of skin cancer are exceptionally responsive to treatment, often requiring no more than a simple excision.

How do I get clients to engage in self-care? In other words, how do we get clients to do their homework? Mostly by not making it seem like homework, and by making it easy to do. When I first started, I wanted to give my clients everything that I learned in my sports massage course, along with a self-massage routine using a lacrosse ball, and a hundred little tips. I imagine some clients left my office feeling a little overwhelmed, and I wouldn't be surprised if it ended up driving some people away. Others might have stayed away because, "I can't go back, I didn't do my homework!"

So, avoid that situation for two reasons: It's needlessly burdensome, and it doesn't work. By keeping your self-care recommendations brief, doable, and easily comprehensible, you'll increase the odds of implementation by about a million percent. That sounds something like this: "Here's a quick stretch I'd like you to try at work. It's something you can do when you feel your upper back starting to get cranky, or every time you get up to go to the bathroom. First, clasp your hands behind your back..." Notice how I gave them a reason to try it, and then suggested a way that they could work it into their existing routine. This is much better than a client learning a stretch but not knowing when to do it or why.

I also recommend saying something like this: "Now, this isn't homework, so don't feel compelled. Just give it a try when and if you feel like it." I say this for a slightly manipulative reason: I've found my clients are *more* likely to try a suggestion when there's not a lot of pressure piled on top of it. This is true for me as well — I base this strategy on a past therapist explicitly telling me, "If you don't do any journaling, don't worry about it. I won't be mad, and you don't have to feel like a student who didn't do their homework." For whatever reason, this completely pressure-free environment helped me find my motivation and actually get the task done. And on weeks when I didn't? I knew it wouldn't be a big deal.

Even if you don't give specific homework, remember that you can act as a general wellness cheerleader. If your client mentions wanting to try yoga? Yeah, that would be cool! It has excellent results for pain reduction in the literature. They want to add running to their regimen? Great idea! Thinking about trying physical therapy? That could really help knock out the last of this pain! Basically, be ready to talk about different ways of approaching pain, be encouraging about new things and experimentation, and send the message that, no matter what, you're in their corner.

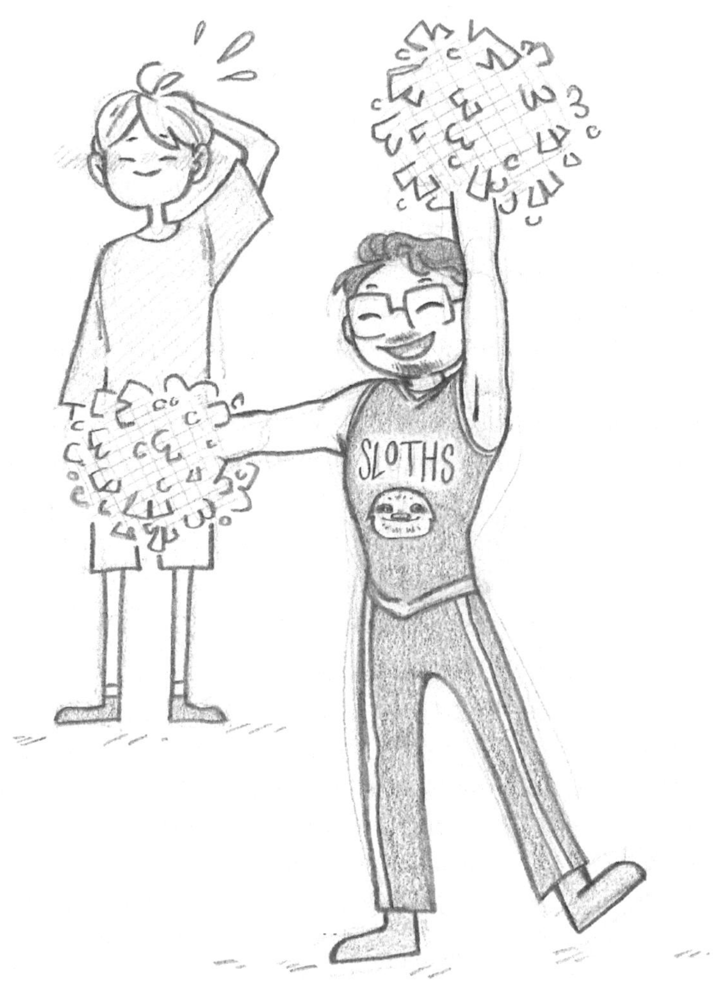

Is giving homework within my scope of practice? This question could be asked about recommending stretches or exercises, using orthopedic testing, or offering certain types of massage. Are you allowed to do so, and is doing so ethical?

The most important thing to note is that this might be directly addressed by your local laws and massage board regulations. They might define your scope comprehensively, leaving little leeway to do things like recommend exercise. In this case, follow the rules in place and consider referring out to well-qualified personal trainers and physical/occupational therapists when additional activity would help.

If your role is less strictly defined, then I say expand outward as your training dictates. In other words, only recommend stretches if you've taken some classes that feature them (sports massage workshops are great for picking up some techniques here), and if you feel confident enough in their application to teach them. Be wary of expanding your treatments or homework so much that you're taking on the role of a personal trainer (or esthetician, or nutritionist) – keep these tangential recommendations well-focused and relevant.

I personally draw the line when it comes to what clients consume or the shape of their body. I don't give diet advice, and I don't recommend supplements, despite extensive experience with both. I can't know their blood chemistry or how their liver processes different compounds, so it would be unwise for me to recommend magnesium for sleep or anxiety. I don't know their relationship with weight gain or weight loss, any trauma they might have relating to these topics, or any underlying medical conditions that might complicate these matters, so I don't talk about dieting. And... I'm a massage therapist! I want them to feel safe in my office, and part of that is sticking to the foundation of massage as my primary form of treatment and the basis of our therapeutic relationship. When they step into my office, they know they won't be hit by a surprise curveball about the supplement I'd like them to try or the essential oil sales group I'd like them to join.

Be a source of sound advice about the body and how to use it, and give homework when it's useful and appropriate. But, first and foremost, let massage be your medicine.

Lightning round!

Why do clients' stomachs growl during massage? The relaxation response! Activation of the parasympathetic nervous system tells the abdominal contents to do their digestion thing via the vagus nerve. This leads to borborygmus (tummy rumbling, which is mostly gas bubbling in the intestines due to increased motility) and sometimes flatulence. This is normal, and it's such a good indicator of relaxation that it might as well be a round of applause.

Why do clients' noses get stuffy during massage? Gravity! Being completely face-down causes blood to pool in the erectile mucosa in the client's nasal cavity. No, it's not caused by the face cradle, and no, it's not mucus build-up that can be solved by blowing the nose (though nasal congestion can lead to more mucus production). The best solution is to change the position of the client's head — have them turn it to the side if they're stuffy and can do so comfortably — or simply have congestion-prone clients spend less time face-down.

Should I offer my client water after a massage? Yep. They'll have dry mouth after getting stuffy and subsequently breathing through their mouth. No, I don't think there are any toxins they need to flush.

What should I do when a client gets an erection? You're usually safe to ignore it completely. Most men will be somewhat embarrassed, and others will know that it's not something under their control. You can use a heavy blanket to keep such things out of sight and out of mind. If someone apologizes, this *can* be a strategy to get you to pay more attention to it, or it can be someone genuinely horrified by the behavior of their own body. The best response here is to reassure while also closing the discussion down: "No worries, it's just one of those things the body does. Now, I'm going to sink in here, go ahead and take some easy, deep breaths..."

(that last part is optional, but it can be a useful strategy to redirect from unwanted conversation back to the massage). If they follow up with other probing questions, you can say, "it's not something I'd like us to dwell on."

What if the erection bounces? That's a voluntary contraction of the pubococcygeal muscles. They're doing a Kegel exercise on purpose, and it's their way of trying to draw your attention to the situation, or a form of self-stimulation. They're being weird and they know it, so boot 'em.

How do I handle hair on the head that I'm not familiar with? Whether it's braids, locs, extensions, a weave, a wig, a beard, or a head covering: Ask, but keep it strictly massage related. "I see you've got your hair styled/covered and I was wondering about scalp massage. Is that something you'd like to skip over or can I work with this area?" If you've got unrelated questions about hair, realize this can be deeply personal (and sometimes even related to religious practice), and Google is a better resource than an in-person interrogation. Oh, and never get oil in someone's hair without asking.

Why do clients feel loopy (or "drunk" or "high") after a massage? There's no clinical research on this, but based on the euphoric qualities and the feeling of being in an altered state, I'd guess (and it's just a guess!) that endocannabinoids and/or endorphins are involved. I've got no reason to believe that these clients are in an impaired state, but it could still be nice to invite them to sit and drink some water or tea before getting behind the wheel.

Chapter 12. Bringing It All Back Together

If you take nothing else away from this book, I'm hoping you'll hang on to these bits and pieces:

1. **Strive for satisfaction, not perfection**. Realize that being "good enough" can be good enough, and indeed it can create a truly amazing experience for clients. Trying to be perfect can lead to *grasping* behaviors, which are almost always a form of self-sabotage.
2. **Focus on the process and let go of outcomes**. Communicate well, offer your attention and your skill, and be mindful as you work. That's all you can control, so put your focus there. Let the outcomes take care of themselves.
3. **Remember the continuum of massage intensity**. Start with what's friendliest to the nervous system because that can be all it takes to reduce pain. Introduce more intense or invasive strategies as needed, and only with the client's robust informed consent.
4. **Don't let fear determine your therapeutic style**. That includes fear of intimacy, fear of certain body parts, or fear of men with bad intentions. Be boldly yourself, communicate thoroughly, and trust that you can enforce your boundaries.
5. **Train like an athlete**. That means cross-training, strengthening yourself in ways that make your job easier, and getting enough rest and relaxation.
6. **Remember the tipping point**. Find promotional strategies that produce small gains (i.e., an extra client per month), and have faith that these will culminate in big dividends.
7. **Sales can be simple**. Tell the client what's true (e.g., "I think it would benefit you to start with weekly massage until these headaches become less frequent"), and then wait. Don't add disclaimers or self-sabotaging apologies — just state your

clinical reasoning, and then let the client decide. The outcome will be the outcome.

8. **Remember the power differential**. Open the floodgates of communication wide, let the client know that they're the expert in the room when it comes to their body, and don't trust polite or deferential answers. If the client says the pressure is "fine," ask a follow-up question.
9. **Recognize dehumanizing elements in your work environment**. Look for aspects of your work that say, "you are a machine," and change them at all costs. Seek community and follow your curiosity.
10. **Remember the tug-of-war**. When you're strategizing about how to work with pain, broaden your focus to all the muscles that might be involved. If a posterior muscle is in pain, think of the anterior muscles that it might be fighting with. Think of the synergists and stabilizers that are part of that web. Think locally, and act globally.

Daily affirmations

I'd like to offer you an affirmation. This is something you can say to yourself when you notice that your mind is in a loop, or you're trying to read a client's mind and worried about them judging you or hating the massage, or if you're just catastrophizing in general. I stole it from the internet[37].

"What if things work out?"

I like this because it's not an absolute statement of belief (i.e., "things will work out"), which are pretty easy to dismiss in an anxious mind. Instead, it's simply a hypothetical that redirects you from catastrophe to a nascent form of faith. Sure, things are rough right now, but they've usually worked out in the past. What if they work out this time, too? Can I sit with that idea for a while, and allow myself to see that future?

---

[37] https://twitter.com/Sinclair_Ceasar/status/983876811523280896

Here's a bonus affirmation for when you're having a hard day: "This is the best damn massage I've ever given. Truly this is the massage of the gods. Witness me and my incredible massage powers!" Basically, counter negative self-talk with bombastic, ridiculous humor, and let yourself smile.

Embrace the weirdness

In this book, I've talked a lot about potentially awkward and difficult subjects. Dealing with intimacy, communicating effectively, and beating burnout. Even the business topics can be pretty anxiety-provoking, requiring you to take repeated leaps of faith as you try new things and face new challenges. As you traverse these unfamiliar landscapes, realize that you can always do so with the same sense of curiosity and playfulness that you bring to massage. Nothing here is punishing, not even taxes — if you screw up, the worst thing that will happen is having to pay back taxes and a reasonable penalty. You don't get publicly flogged or shot out of a cannon.

So, as you ask yourself, "what if things work out," you can also ask, "what if I have fun with this?" Recognize that communication and business, and even pain relief and massage strategy, are all inherently forgiving. Massage is pizza, nobody will remember your "ums" and verbal missteps, and if you forget to submit a form, some bureaucrat will let you know.

Massage is weird. We're healthcare professionals, we're artists, we're healers, we're cheerleaders. We'll see a client with low back pain in the morning, a client with anxiety in the afternoon, and a client on a spiritual journey to close out the day, and that's just an average Tuesday.

Embrace the weirdness and realize that you always have a stable foundation to return to: Your breath. No matter what you're facing, no matter what big task you've got coming up, no matter how much your next client tends to stress you out, you can always choose to set all that aside, and just breathe.

You can try it with me here if you like. To begin, just take some easy, slow breaths, allowing them to be slightly deeper than usual.

Shift your mind's eye to your abdominal muscles and see if you can allow them to soften. As you breathe in, you might notice your belly poke out, and that's okay. It's great, in fact.

Now, pay a moment's attention to your mind. Did you notice anything shift as you tried that simple, one-step exercise? You might notice a slight decrease in mental tension, and maybe the things you were stressed out about suddenly seem a little further away, a little less immediate.

This is something that you can share with your clients as well. Invite them to take some easy, deep breaths as you work with a significant area. Invite them to allow their abdominal muscles to soften and poke out. They can imagine their breath traveling to the area under your hands, softening it and warming it, and allowing it to melt. As they breathe, you can join them, allowing your breath to synchronize with theirs. See if you can imagine what it's like in their body, and what the sensation is like under your hands. Eventually, you might find that all you need to do to invite your clients to deepen their breathing is for you to take some deep breaths yourself.

Realize that your breath is always there, always going in and out like the waves of an ocean. Any time you find yourself stuck in a loop of self-deprecation or catastrophizing or fear, slow your breathing, allow it to deepen, and take a mental step back. Don't feel like this is a moral imperative, or the way you "should" breathe — rather, this is a tool you can use to reconnect with your body when you'd otherwise be stuck in your head.

An ode to stillness

During your next massage, there's something I'd like you to try. Take one of those million feel-good techniques that you know, apply it to a feel-good area of the body, and then... stop.

Grasp the traps, and then just hold them for a while. Sink pressure over the ischial tuberosity, and then just hang out. Find a comfortable way to cradle the skull, and then don't move a muscle for a full thirty seconds.

Imagine being a client and your therapist finds that perfect spot, and then just stops. For the next ten breaths, you get to really experience that part of your body, perhaps for the first time in your life. You get to connect with your SI joint, which you had never really been aware of before. You get to experience your infraspinatus muscle, which had always felt like an undifferentiated part of your back.

Stillness, paradoxically, is a conversation. It invites communion between the client and their own body. It gives a chance for the spinal cord to realize that the default resting tone doesn't need to be so high, and for the brain to dial down its sensitivity. All without moving a muscle or gliding an inch.

Static contacts aren't the "right" way to do massage, or the only way. I bring them up in this last chapter because I want you to remember that they exist. Stillness feels great, it's profound, and it's easy. Collect those tools that are easy and effective, and let them sit at the top of your toolbox.

Remember the whole person

When you're working with a client, remember that they're a whole person, an entire world made up of years and decades of complicated life experience. There is so much to learn from each of them, and so much to teach in return. If you find yourself reducing a client to parts, take a mental step back and remind yourself of how each person is endlessly interconnected. Bring that spirit into your massage and use your hands to remind the client of their wholeness.

If you find yourself reducing clients to numbers, or to good clients and bad clients, to ideal and problematic, take a step back from that reductive thinking. Labels are a way of reducing cognitive load so that you can more easily categorize and respond to the world around you. When it comes to people, throw labels out the window and choose to see the complexity in front of you.

Do the same for yourself. You are a person, a world of philosophy and history, trials and triumphs. You are worthy of consideration, love, and kindness.

That's it.

That's everything I know about massage, all written down in one place. I hope you weren't interested in a sequel because this is all I got. It took me six years, I hit a lot of plateaus and roadblocks, I got to experience writer's block (burnout!), and I needed a good psychologist to help me get out of my own way and just write. But I got there in the end. I'm grateful to you for joining me.

Massage is weird. I may have mentioned that a few times. Every technique that we use, every modality — they're all made up. Someone mashed or squeezed tissue in a specific way, other people iterated on that approach, and eventually we had Swedish massage. Modern day teachers and gurus come up with new systems on a daily basis, give them sciencey-sounding names, and the next generation sees that as received wisdom. But y'all, if they can make things up, so can you. You can be your own modality, you can try interesting new ways of approaching the body, and you can call it whatever you want. Be free of dogma and prescriptivism. Be formless, shapeless, like water.

And mostly, have fun. Massage isn't serious business. There is no such thing as a massage emergency, and any client or boss who tells you otherwise is wrong. Yes, it can be a powerful approach to pain and a useful adjunct to a wellness routine, but we're not cardiac surgeons. We're not mission control for a rocket launch, or air traffic controllers. We're tissue squishers! Enjoy yourself, dance in your studio, try something new every day.

Be the rolling pebble that starts the landslide of self-care that finally gets people out of chronic pain. Be a wellness cheerleader, and your client's most fervent advocate. Make powerful connections in the context of well-defined boundaries, and watch how those flowers bloom.

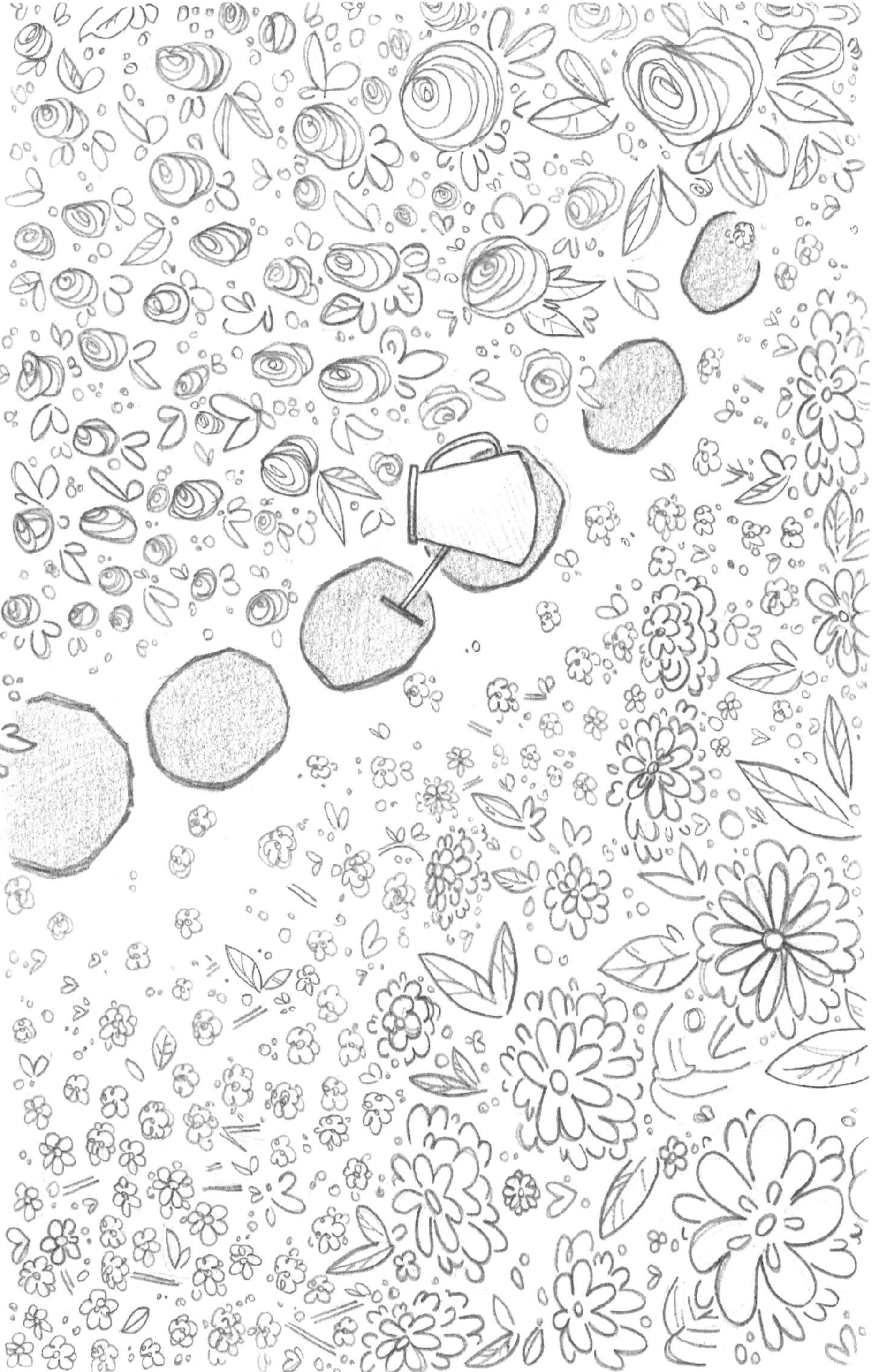

My Workshop

If you've made it this far, you might be interested in the workshop that I teach. It's called "Myofascial Swedish," and it's a two-day, 16-hour, NCBTMB-approved continuing education class for massage therapists of all experience levels. We spend a full day connecting with the fascia, by which I mean working broadly and throwing our weight around. We experiment with stillness, and play with lots of fun hand placements. On day two, we take those principles and apply them to a slow, flowing, landslide style of massage. It's a good thing. You can find more information at massagesloth.com/myofascialswedish/ (and make sure to sign up for the mailing list to stay up to date).

And while I've got you here, I'd love for you to review this book on Amazon. A couple of sentences about how it applied to you and your practice could help newcomers determine whether it's worth their while.

See what I did there? Shaping the kinds of reviews I get? I literally can't turn it off.

Acknowledgements:

Beta Readers:
Samantha Andrews
Ian Brown
Rebecca Fisher
Christine McLean
Karen Paavola
Julianna Parlock
Beth Patton
Jeff Phelps
Anne Reilly
Emily White
Anna Wong

My deepest thanks to all my beta readers and cheerleaders. To everyone who ever sent me a question or reached out because they thought they were alone in their doubts and fears. To everyone on the Massage Sloth Clubhouse (it's a forum! Search for it on Facebook and join us) for being a source of inspiration. To my family, who always has my back.